THE HOT LATIN DIET

THE
HOT

THE FAST-TRACK PLAN

LATIN

TO A BOMBSHELL BODY

DIET

Dr. Manny Alvarez

WITH ARLEN GARGAGLIANO

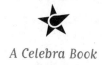

A Celebra Book

Celebra
Published by New American Library, a division of
Penguin Group (USA) Inc., 375 Hudson Street,
New York, New York 10014, USA.
Penguin Group (Canada), 90 Eglinton Avenue East, Suite 700, Toronto,
Ontario M4P 2Y3, Canada (a division of Pearson Penguin Canada Inc.).
Penguin Books Ltd., 80 Strand, London WC2R 0RL, England
Penguin Ireland, 25 St. Stephen's Green, Dublin 2,
Ireland (a division of Penguin Books Ltd.).
Penguin Group (Australia), 250 Camberwell Road, Camberwell, Victoria 3124,
Australia (a division of Pearson Australia Group Pty. Ltd.).
Penguin Books India Pvt. Ltd., 11 Community Centre, Panchsheel Park,
New Delhi - 110 017, India.
Penguin Group (NZ), 67 Apollo Drive, Rosedale, North Shore 0632,
New Zealand (a division of Pearson New Zealand Ltd.).
Penguin Books (South Africa) (Pty.) Ltd., 24 Sturdee Avenue,
Rosebank, Johannesburg 2196, South Africa

Penguin Books Ltd., Registered Offices:
80 Strand, London WC2R 0RL, England

First published by Celebra,
a division of Penguin Group (USA) Inc.

First Printing, May 2008
10 9 8 7 6 5 4 3 2 1

For photo credits, see page 204.

CELEBRA and logo are trademarks of Penguin Group (USA) Inc.

LIBRARY OF CONGRESS CATALOGING-IN-PUBLICATION DATA:

Alvarez, Manny.
The hot latin diet: the fast-track plan to a bombshell body/Manny Alvarez with Arlen Gargagliano.
p.   cm.
ISBN 978-0-451-22371-5
1. Reducing diets.   2. Cookery, Latin American.   3. Women—Health and hygiene.   I. Gargagliano, Arlen.   II. Title.
RM222.2.A456 2008
613.2'5—dc22   2007045341

Set in Matrix Book
Designed by Liney Li

Printed in the United States of America

PUBLISHER'S NOTE

Every effort has been made to ensure that the information contained in this book is complete and accurate. However, neither the publisher nor the author is engaged in rendering professional advice or services to the individual reader. The ideas, procedures, and suggestions contained in this book are not intended as a substitute for consulting with your physician. All matters regarding your health require medical supervision. Neither the author nor the publisher shall be liable or responsible for any loss or damage allegedly arising from any information or suggestion in this book. The opinions expressed in this book represent the personal views of the author and not of the publisher.

The recipes contained in this book are to be followed exactly as written. The publisher is not responsible for your specific health or allergy needs that may require medical supervision. The publisher is not responsible for any adverse reactions to the recipes contained in this book.

The publisher does not have any control over and does not assume any responsibility for author or third-party Web sites or their content.

To my wife, Katarina, and children, Rex, Ryan and Olivia.

With you always.

ACKNOWLEDGMENTS

I would like to express my sincere appreciation and gratitude to the staff at Penguin Group. Their tremendous support is what inspires me to continue writing. I would especially like to thank my publisher, Raymond Garcia, who always makes sure I cross my t's and dot my i's. Of course I could not have written this book alone; I had a lot of help, especially from all the wonderful chefs; they are a true collection of talent and grace. I also need to thank our great nutritionist, Kena Custage, for her wonderful analysis and advice. My words would have been lost if not for the help of Arlen Gargagliano, one of the best writers who truly understands the art of cooking.

Finally let's not forget the people who have contributed to, and continue to contribute to, my success: Roger Ailes, for being a true friend and for guiding me through his advice and making "health" an important part of FOX News. The staff at Hackensack University Medical Center; from physicians to nurses, the best in the world! To my inner circle—Haydee Mato, Dr. Al-Khan, Mike Petriella, Mildred Espinosa. And of course my family in New Jersey and Florida—thank you for keeping me out of trouble.

Most of all, I thank you, the reader. I hope that when you get through this book, you will be as enchanted as I have always been with the beauty of the Latin culture, its tradition, emotion, and of course, its "salsa."

Always thinking of you,
Dr. Manny

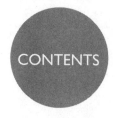

CONTENTS

THE HOT LATIN DIET

INTRODUCTION

O*ne of the reasons I came up with the Hot Latin Diet* has a lot to do with being an ob-gyn for over thirty years. Throughout my career, I've had hundreds of mommies—and soon-to-be-moms—coming through my office door. What I've noticed is that over the past few decades, moms have been gaining significant weight during their pregnancies, and then they haven't lost that weight—in fact, they have gotten heavier after just two years. We've seen an epidemic of obesity in children and type 2 diabetes in females. The rules for pregnancy weight gain have had to change; we used to say gain twenty-five to thirty pounds during pregnancy, but today most moms start overweight, so these numbers have dropped to an average of twenty to twenty-five pounds. I try to help moms limit their excess weight gain, but this is tough. What this tells me is that we've gotten out of control with eating in this country—and that is true not just for women, but for all of us.

I am disturbed by the alarming growth (yes, literally!!) of the entire American population. The statistics speak for themselves: chronic diseases (cardiovascular disease, cancer, and diabetes) are now among the most prevalent, costly, and preventable of all health problems, yet they affect the lives of more than 90 million Americans (not to mention the cost of health care); 1.7 million people die annually as a result of chronic disease, which translates into the deaths of seven out of ten people. And despite the fact that chronic diseases are perhaps the most common and costly of health problems, they are also among the most preventable. They can simply be prevented by what we put in our mouths.

In addition to studying the eating habits of people in the United States, I have also noticed that most families who immigrate from the Caribbean Basin and other points of Latin America are fit and trim when they arrive in the United States; however, if you look at this same community three years later, they're usually overweight. I've experienced this with patients time and time again. I know of one little girl, for example, who moved with her parents from the Dominican Republic. She arrived here at age twelve as a perfectly fit prepubescent teen. Now this girl is eighteen years old, and weighs three hundred pounds. What happened?

Well, what happened to this girl is indicative of what happens to so many of us in America: we're bombarded by marketing that presents us with foods that we "must" have, when, in reality, they're not the right choices; we live in a fast-paced society that discourages good habits and priorities like walking, exercising, and even relaxing, and most important, this fast-paced lifestyle has led to the desire for fast food, which doesn't just mean McDonald's anymore. Today's fast foods are also meal bars, on-the-go shakes, and prepackaged foods, which contain high levels of sodium and preservatives that wear down our muscle tissue, slow down our metabolism, make us gain weight, and may even shorten our life span.

We can look back not too long ago to see how we've all changed in terms of our relationship with food and fitness. When my parents were young, life was very different; their priorities and focuses were also different—food was essential and respected, activity was part of work and daily life, and home cooking with natural ingredients was the norm. Today, our time is very limited and there has been a shift in priorities and goals—while food is essential, it's not so respected, activity is modest, and eating out or eating packaged meals has become the norm. What we need to do is return to the outlook that food—and activity—is essential; this is the way we can eliminate the many fatalities caused by disease, increase our feeling of well-being and energy, and live a longer and better life. We need to get back to our parents' approach!

Determined to address my patients' weight issues and our country's booming increase in preventable disease, and inspired by the positive things I saw growing up, I went back to examine my own culinary roots, and as a Cuban American, those of my Latino brethren. I was amazed to find high levels of life expectancy and low levels of obesity in a culture almost defined by its food. I was also surprised to find that many Miss Universe winners are actually of Latin American heritage— the same winners who claim to "never diet." I knew that there had to be an underlying common thread in our diet to explain this, and I was resolved to unearth the key ingredients and factors associated with this remarkably healthy lifestyle. After careful study, what I discovered became the backbone to this diet and the source of a healthy lifestyle:

The Seven Latin Powerfoods

tomatillos

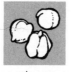
garbanzo beans

avocado

garlic

cinnamon

chiles

cilantro

The nutritional and antioxidant components found in the seven Latin powerfoods will help your body become strong and nourished. Incorporating these foods into your diet will also help you feel full while staying healthy. You'll quickly start to notice how you no longer feel heavy and sluggish after meals—instead you'll find that you have more energy than before! Overall, the three major benefits of these powerfoods are that they help your body:

1. function at an optimal level by flushing out the toxins from your cells, allowing them to operate more efficiently;

2. enhance metabolic function, speeding up weight loss;

3. boost key fat-burning vessels—adding strength, muscle mass, power, and stamina.

The Hot Latin Diet is the first plan to unveil the top seven Latin powerfoods, helping you to include them in your everyday life. This diet is built on the foundation of one of the most basic of Latin philosophies: Life must be enjoyed! Therefore, quality of life is a huge consideration in this diet. Of course, quality includes probably the most fundamental component: eating well. In fact, I'm not going to tell you to take fat completely out of your diet; I can't live without my olive oil—and a few others! (Okay, sometimes many others. . . .) But I will say that it's all about balance (and totally *not* about excess). This means great culinary variety—with depth of flavor, including plenty of spice (and I'm not talking hot! I'm talking taste!). Deprivation, unhappiness, and disappointment—especially with oneself—do not enter into this realm of thinking.

The seven Latin powerfoods are also bursting with flavor and full of the nutrients your body craves and needs. Having these powerfoods at your disposal also means great culinary variety. The Latin American diet is now a brilliant amalgam of many different cultures and ingredients. With millions of immigrants from Latin America (including Mexico and Brazil) and the Caribbean, we've been blessed here in the States (and Canada) with a plethora of foods and ingredients that even as recently as fifteen years ago couldn't be found in our markets. What's happening today in the Latin American food world is that we're getting the best of the best! We're sharing our culinary secrets—and the results, as you can see by my recipes, are a combination of fabulously flavorful and healthful ingredients.

Now I didn't create these recipes and this diet alone. These wonderful recipes were contributed by the world-renowned Latina chefs Xiomara Ardolina, Michelle Bernstein, Daisy Martínez, Zarela Martínez, and Sue Torres. In addition, Kena Custage, a board-certified nutritionist and holistic health practitioner (as well as a licensed psychotherapist, breath and meditation therapist, and Reiki master) was instrumental in designing these meals and charts, as well as providing all the accompanying nutritional advice. Finally, I wrote this book along with chef Arlen Gargagliano. She inherited her passion for food from her mom and honed her skills with the Colombian-born chef Rafael Palomino, whom she's worked with for the past twelve years. These women are all amazing! They're as talented as they are passionate about their craft. What I hope you'll get from these chefs is not only inspiration but also many, many ideas. As you look through their recipes, you'll discover different ways of combining ingredients, foods, and spices in your everyday life.

I will also tell you this from the start: the Hot Latin Diet is not a fad. Most people in this country are obsessed with losing weight and with diets promising to help them shed pounds in mere weeks. Sure, they might work at first, but the reality is that most people quickly gain those pounds back. Why? Because most of these diets are fads. What they don't teach you is that losing weight isn't just about a diet change and following the motions; it is, instead, about lifestyle changes.

I know that getting started is often the hardest part, so here's what I'm suggesting. First, since you've obviously made the decision that there are going to be some changes in your life (which, I hope you realize, is one of the biggest decisions of all!), you need to remember that any change should happen slowly: one bite at a time, if you will. But even now you need to remember to be patient with yourself. Second, read this book one time through, so that you have an idea of what steps you need to take, and how you'll get there. Third, keep coming back for more! You should go back and consult pages that you've already read, for both information and support.

Not only will I be giving you general suggestions and tips, I'll also be giving you specific ones based on your age group. In my book *The Checklist*, I outlined what you and your family need to know, according to each decade of your life, to live long and healthy lives. Here I'm going to give you specifically tailored instructions to help you do the same—but based on your diet. But remember, if you really want to lose weight, you have to do two things: eat fewer calories and burn more calories.

The goal of this book is to inform and motivate you. There's a lot of information here, and you can't possibly absorb it all at once. As you know, inspiration is not a one-shot deal, so I encourage you to go back and find the information that most stimulated you into moving toward your goal (and it's *my* goal to furnish you with a lot of tools that you can reach for when you need that extra push to keep on going and following your dreams). Finally, find what works for you, and keep at it. Again, it's all about balance: feeling good always leads to looking good.

In our quest for balance, it's interesting to me that everyone—myself included—may have a different reason for getting into shape.

Ironically, the main reason, being healthy, doesn't seem to be in the forefront. Some reasons you may recognize are:

- ▶ Vanity—You want to look better! You want to wear a cocktail dress (and look like you should be wearing it), or not be embarrassed in a bathing suit, or shorts, or anything you'd like to wear.

- ▶ Changing a particular area (or several areas!) of your body—legs, hips, chin(s)—because they're too big or bulky as they are right now. You want them narrower, stronger, leaner, and meaner!

- ▶ Making someone else happy—You know your significant other likes you a bit slimmer, or you want your kids to be proud of you, or you want that cute guy across the hall to pay more attention to you.

Whatever your reasons are, I want you to consider something. The Hot Latin Diet is a lifestyle change. This is going to be different from what you've done before, and it's going to help you achieve your weight goal—regardless of your motivation. However, I would also like to contribute to your understanding of the importance of the health reason, and remind you—as I'll continue to do—that if you feel better, my friend, because of a new diet, new exercise, and your new attitude, you will look better. But before we move forward, I have a request: I want you to make a commitment to focus on the new.

In a nutshell, the Hot Latin Diet is a base for a long, happy, and healthy life. This book will teach you how to incorporate the seven Latin powerfoods into your everyday diet, the reasons behind weight gain and how to prevent it, and how to set your weight-loss goals and achieve them, not only for a summer, but for life.

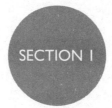

SECTION I

THE HOT LATIN DIET

- ☑ *Details on the Seven Latin Powerfoods*

- ☑ *The Seven Latin Powerfood Categories*

- ☑ *The Hot Latin Diet Versus Other Diets*

- ☑ *Why the Hot Latin Diet?*

- ☑ *Making the Hot Latin Diet Work for You*

- ☑ *How to Execute the Plan*

Details on the Seven Latin Powerfoods

By eating the seven Latin powerfoods, by ingesting foods with antioxidant properties, and by eliminating bad oils and implementing good ones, you're detoxifying yourself. What does this mean? Well, basically, every human cell takes food, burns it, creates waste, and then discards it. We all generate cellular by-products. However, when the cell doesn't get rid of waste, we become less efficient. And when the waste is contaminated, it is difficult to eliminate. What we want is to have our cells metabolize effectively. Toxins don't allow cells to work well. In order for us to lose weight, our cells must be working well. That's why antioxidants, proteins, and good oils become important when you start to talk dieting and health. That's also why when we see news reports about lowering cancer rates, they're always—if you notice—linked with balanced diets. At the end of the day, cancers, aside from being genetically derived, are derived from cellular toxicity from poor diets and habits (like smoking and drinking).

The good news about all this is that you can eliminate a lot of the toxins in your body—and your body will respond relatively quickly. Consider this example using one of the most toxic activities people do to themselves: smoke. Did you know that if you quit smoking—even after twenty years of doing it—your body will immediately change? In fact, even after one hour of not smoking, the oxygen content in your cells is significantly higher! Now if your body responds that quickly to stopping one of the most detrimental toxins from invading it, you can recognize that a change in the body's diet is also going to have immediate, beneficial effects.

Let's look further into the seven Latin powerfoods and their subcategories and learn about their immediate effects on our bodies.

TOMATILLOS

These flavorful and unique small yellow-green tomatoes pack a lot more nutrients than regular red tomatoes. Used throughout Mexico and available now here in the States, tomatillos are rich in vitamins C, A, and folic acid, as well as potassium. They are a great source for your daily antioxidant needs.

GARBANZO BEANS

These delicious beans are very high in fiber, which will improve your elimination cycles and support the growth of healthy intestinal flora. They are very low in natural sugar content, and high in complex carbohydrate content and protein, giving you a steady source of high-quality fuel for balanced energy throughout your day. They also have a warming effect on your body and a calming effect on your mind. Garbanzo beans are used in cooking throughout Latin America and the Caribbean.

AVOCADO

Do not let the "high" fat content of avocados deter you from eating this fantastic fruit. In fact, the healthy monounsaturated oil in avocado will help you feel satiated after a meal and signal your body to burn more fat stores, as well as lower your bad cholesterol and raise your good cholesterol! Avocado also helps lubricate your intestines and assists in regulating your elimination cycles. Avocados are grown, and consumed, throughout the Americas.

GARLIC

Use garlic as often as you can in your cooking. Garlic is well known for its immune-boosting and antimicrobial properties. It also helps lower bad cholesterol. A clove of garlic a day can keep the doctor away! You will benefit from improved blood circulation as well as a stronger libido. The Spanish, Portuguese, and French are credited with introducing this powerfood to the New World, where it is now a ubiquitous ingredient.

CINNAMON

A half teaspoon a day of cinnamon can lower sugar levels in your blood, and studies show that cinnamon can aid in the prevention of diabetes. Cinnamon is also high in antioxidants, not to mention flavor. You can sprinkle cinnamon on fruits or whole grains instead of sugar for a delicious treat. You will also benefit from its sensually warming and cholesterol-lowering qualities. First used medicinally in Egypt and India and in parts of Europe since about 500 BC, this spice is now part of many Latin American and Caribbean cuisines.

CHILES

You can use chiles as often as you wish in your dishes for flavor and for health. Chiles of all types, like chipotle and other hot chiles, are high in minerals and antioxidants, giving a healthy boost to your immune system. Another interesting note about this powerfood is that although it is hot to taste, it actually has a cooling effect on your body. Blood rushes to the periphery of your body in response to the hot taste, and then the blood cools down before moving more to the center of your body, where your temperature is higher. That is why Latinos in hot tropical countries instinctively eat hot and spicy foods. Though many equate chiles with Mexico, they can be found in varied colors and shapes, as well as all different degrees of hotness, throughout Latin America and the Caribbean.

CILANTRO

Cilantro accelerates the excretion of toxic metals from your body. Excess toxic metals in the body can create a breeding ground for viral infections, so using cilantro on a daily basis in your cooking is a very smart choice for staying healthy. All you need is a handful in a salad or a couple of tablespoons in a cooked dish to reap the benefits of this medicinal plant. This herb—and its cousin, culantro—is used throughout the Americas.

Aside from these seven Latin powerfoods, there is a great assortment of others that fall under the same categories. These powerfoods contain a myriad of options offering benefits similar to the ones I've mentioned. If you're looking for more variety—which is one of the main advantages of following a Latin diet—look at the powerfood categories below. You'll see where each of the seven Latin powerfoods falls within the food groups and what other similar foods you can work with. Be creative! More color means more nutrients. By combining these healthy and natural Latin ingredients, you'll be sure to optimize their effects!

(1) **Beans:** garbanzos (chickpeas), lentils, black beans, red kidney beans, and pinto beans.

(2) **Fruits:** mangoes, papayas, pineapples, cherimoyas, passion fruit, guavas, limes, and the Brazilian berry açaí.

(3) **Vegetables and chiles:** tomatoes, plantains, avocados, jícama (Mexican potato or turnip), nopales (prickly pear cactus), calabaza (West Indian pumpkin), jalapeño, chipotle, and more.

④ **Grains, tubers, and nuts:** quinoa, amaranth, yuca (cassava or manioc), yautía, corn, rice, pine nuts, peanuts, and pecans, to name a few.

⑤ **Seafoods:** shrimp, clams, snapper, the eel-like congrio, trout, and sea bass.

⑥ **Poultry:** free-range organic chicken, turkey, quail (and eggs!), and more.

⑦ **Meat:** principally organic beef, lamb, and pork.

The Seven Latin Powerfood Categories

BEANS	Serving	Calories	Total Fat	Carbs.	Fiber	Sugars	Protein	Antioxidant Rating
garbanzos	**1 cup cooked**	**207**	**3.4g**	**34.4g**	**9.9g**	**1.1g**	**11g**	**1**
lentils	1 cup cooked	201	0.6g	34.1g	17.3g	1.2g	14.7g	1
black beans	1 cup cooked	227	0.9g	40.8g	15g	0	15.2g	2
red kidney beans	1 cup cooked	197	0	35.8g	10.7g	3.6g	14.3g	5
pinto beans	1 cup cooked	206	1g	36.6g	11g	0.5g	11.7g	5

Note: All beans are cholesterol-free, and ⅓ cup dry beans equals 1 cup cooked. The higher the antioxidant rating (which is based on the ORAC, or Oxygen Radical Absorbance Capacity, scale; this is a method gauging antioxidant power), the more that food will help you. Garbanzo beans are a powerfood to be enjoyed often!

FRUIT	Serving	Calories	Total Fat	Carbs.	Fiber	Sugars	Protein	Antioxidant Rating
mango	I cup	107	0.4g	28.1g	3.0g	24.4g	0.8g	2
papaya	I cup	59	0.2g	14.9g	2.7g	9g	0.9g	I
pineapple	I cup	113	0.3g	29.8g	3.3g	21.7g	1.3g	2
cherimoya	I cup	116	0.9g	28g	3.6g	2.7g	0	3
passion fruit	I cup	122	0.2g	27g	2.9g	14g	1.1g	2
guava	I cup	112	0.4g	23.6g	8.9g	14.7g	4.2g	2
açaí	I cup	302	12g	40g	10g	30g	8g	5
lime	I cup	60	0.6g	20.1g	1g	4g	1g	3
orange	I cup	90	0.2g	22.6g	4.6g	18g	1.8g	2
watermelon	I cup	74	0.3g	19.1g	1g	15.4g	1.3g	I
baby bananas	I cup	134	0.2g	34.3g	3.9g	18.3g	1.6g	I

Note: All fruits are cholesterol-free.

VEGETABLES AND CHILES	Serving	Calories	Total Fat	Carbs.	Fiber	Sugars	Protein	Antioxidant Rating
tomato	I cup	32	0.4g	7.1g	2.2g	4.7g	1.6g	2
tomatillo	**I cup**	**42**	**1.3g**	**7.7g**	**2.5g**	**5.2g**	**1.3g**	**2**
plantain	I cup	181	0.5g	47g	3.4g	22.2g	1.9g	I
yellow onion	I cup	46	0.1g	11.1g	1.5g	4.7g	1g	3
avocado	**I cup**	**234**	**21.4g**	**12.5g**	**9.8g**	**1g**	**2.9g**	**3**
jícama	I cup	100	0.2g	24g	11g	4g	1.8g	I
nopale	I cup	42	0.5g	9.9g	3.7g	0	0.8g	I
pumpkin	I cup	110	0.2g	29g	4.9g	5.9g	2.9g	3
artichoke	I cup hearts	93	0.3g	20g	10.7g	0	6.5g	5
radish	I cup	19	0.1g	3.9g	1.9g	2.5g	0.8g	I
spinach	I cup	7	0.1g	1.1g	0.7g	0.1g	0.9g	3
red bell pepper	I cup	39	0.4g	9g	3g	6.3g	1.5g	2
jalapeño	**I cup**	**32**	**0**	**2.1g**	**0**	**0**	**0**	**2**
chipotle	**I cup**	**28**	**0**	**2.1g**	**0**	**0**	**0**	**2**

Note: All vegetables and chiles are cholesterol-free. Avocado and hot chiles are powerfoods to be enjoyed often!

GRAINS, TUBERS, NUTS, AND OILS

	Serving	Calories	Total Fat	Carbs.	Fiber	Sugars	Protein	Antioxidant Rating
quinoa	1 cup cooked	254	3.9g	46.9g	4g	0	8.9g	3
amaranth	1 cup cooked	250	4.2g	43.1g	9.7g	1.4g	9.7g	3
brown rice	1 cup cooked	216	1.8g	44.8g	3.5g	0.7g	5g	2
wild rice	1 cup cooked	166	0.6g	35g	3g	1.2g	6.5g	2
corn	1 cup cooked	166	1.1g	40.8g	2.4g	2.9g	2.9g	1
yuca	1 cup boiled	188	0	50.8g	3.8g	1.7g	1.4g	1
malanga/yautía	1 cup cooked	132	0.5g	32g	2g	20g	2g	2
camote/boniato	1 cup cooked	140	0.4g	32.3g	4g	28.3g	2.2g	2
olive oil	1 tablespoon	120	14g	0	0	0	0	1
coconut oil	1 tablespoon	120	14g	0	0	0	0	1
pine nuts	⅓ cup	320	28g	8g	3g	0	13g	2
peanuts	⅓ cup	332	28.2g	12.2g	4.5g	2.4g	13.5g	1
brazil nuts	⅓ cup	381	38.1g	8g	4g	2g	8g	2
pecan nuts	⅓ cup	403	42.2g	7.7g	5.3g	2.3g	5.4g	4

Note: All grains, tubers, nuts, and vegetable oils are cholesterol-free, and ⅓ cup dry grains equals 1 cup cooked. **Nuts can be raw or roasted—raw is healthier.**

SEAFOOD

	Serving	Calories	Total Fat	Cholesterol	Protein
shrimp	6 oz.	169	1.8g	332mg	35.6g
clams	6 oz.	252	3.3g	114mg	43.5g
snapper	6 oz.	218	2.9g	80mg	44.7g
trout	6 oz.	256	9.9g	118mg	39.1g
sea bass	6 oz.	211	4.4g	90mg	40.3g
octopus	6 oz.	279	3.5g	164mg	50.8g

Note: Seafood contains virtually no carbohydrates, sugar, fiber, or antioxidants, and this chart lists cooked portions.

POULTRY AND EGGS	Serving	Calories	Total Fat	Cholesterol	Protein
chicken	6 oz.	281	3.6g	145mg	51g
turkey	6 oz.	322	7g	130mg	54g
quail	6 oz.	375	10g	134mg	42.8g
eggs	3 med.	190	13.2g	554mg	16.4g

Note: Poultry and eggs contain virtually no carbohydrates, sugar, fiber, or antioxidants, and this chart lists cooked portions.

MEAT Lean Cuts	Serving	Calories	Total Fat	Cholesterol	Protein
beef	6 oz.	312	9.9g	99mg	59.9g
lamb	6 oz.	343	16.6g	148mg	45.2g
pork	6 oz.	368	17.1g	138mg	50.2g

Note: Red meats contain virtually no carbohydrates, sugar, fiber, or antioxidants.

Let's look into these categories to understand their true benefits.

BEEF ON BEANS

Beans—a whole host of varieties—have been part of the Latin American diet for centuries. And yes, it's true: Beans are good for your heart! But there's so much more. Beans are extremely beneficial in an antidiabetic diet because they rank low on the glycemic scale—unlike "staples" in the American diet like refined grains and baked goods, which often cause the inflammatory, hunger-inducing spike in blood-sugar levels. They could even help with lowering the risk of colon cancer. Legumes (dried beans and peas) are also a major source of several nutrients—magnesium, potassium, folate, and cholesterol-lowering fiber—most often missing in Americans' diets.

GLORIOUS FRUITS

The fruit bowl is a beautiful thing, especially when it's laden with some of my favorites—pineapples, papayas, and the supersexy mango, or the intoxicatingly wonderful passion fruit. We are so lucky to now have access practically year-round to tropical fruit like the kind I grew up with in my native Cuba. There's a whole wide world of fruit, all with different medicinal and tasty powers. Take cherimoya (the custard apple), for example. This tropical, heart-shaped, dinosaur-skinned fruit has a flesh—and texture—reminiscent of honey, pineapple, and banana. It's an excellent source of vitamin C, a good source of vitamin B$_6$ (which has nerve-calming benefits), as well as calcium, iron, manganese—which helps activate some enzymes—and potassium, which helps regulate blood pressure. Compare that with a bowl of chips! Seriously, as in the case of any kind of eating, variety is key; don't be afraid to try some of those tropical fruit treats.

FROM PLANTAINS TO PUMPKIN

If you're wondering why plantains are in the vegetable section, let me explain: though they look very similar to their cousin the banana, they're actually quite different and act more like potatoes; they must be cooked prior to eating. Throughout Latin America, plantains are more than just wonderful additions to soups and stews. Unlike potatoes, these treats can be used in all stages of ripeness—from green to almost black! Plantains do not contain any cholesterol or sodium and are low in fat. They contain a good dose of calcium, iron, and potassium, are high in vitamin A, and provide an excellent source of fiber.

Pumpkin, another ubiquitous vegetable found throughout Latin America, is also full of taste and health benefits! Whether it's steamed or baked, or added as a flavorful thickener to all kinds of soups and rice and bean dishes, it makes a delicious and healthy addition. Though low in calories, its bright orange flesh is rich in antioxidants and carotenes, as well as potassium and vitamins C and E. It may lower cancer risk, heart attacks, cataracts, and strokes.

GREAT GRAINS

The traditional Latin American diet is filled with so many grains, many of which are just recently making their way up north. Take quinoa, which hails from the Andean region and dates back thousands of years. The Incas were certainly well versed in many areas, nutrition among them. After all, it was the Incas who recognized the stamina-building value in quinoa. In fact, they called it *chisaya mama* (the mother of all grains). This easy-to-prepare and nutritionally well-endowed, almost nut-flavored grain, which has a nice, fluffy texture when cooked, is a healthy and flavorful alternative to white rice. This protein-packed grain is also a very good source of manganese, as well as magnesium, iron, copper, and phosphorous, and may be especially valuable for folks who suffer from migraine headaches, diabetes, and atherosclerosis.

Tubers? Where to begin! Let me start by saying if you've never tried the high-carb, nutty, buttery, and smooth flesh of yuca, then you've been missing a lot! Don't be put off by the barklike outside; this tuber is a fabulous alternative to potatoes.

Nuts are key players on my wife's "yes you can have this as a snack" list! Rich in fiber, and antioxidants, such as vitamin E and selenium, they're a perfect alternative to unhealthy foods when you're craving something satisfying—and fast—to munch on! Nuts are also high in fat, but mostly monounsaturated and polyunsaturated fats, such as omega-3—the good fats—which have all been shown to lower LDL cholesterol (see www.healthcastle.com/nuts-benefits.shtml). Even just lightly toasted (no salt, please!), nuts are a great addition to a leafy green salad, adding both variety of flavor and texture. But please note that the toasted nuts—because the oils are altered in the heating process—won't last as long. Also, keep your fresh nuts in the freezer to give them a longer life.

THE SECRETS OF SEAFOOD

Actually the secret is—as always—freshness and variety! These light white meat and natural ocean feeders (not bottom-feeders) have so many attributes beyond great flavor, whether marinated lightly for a ceviche (a wonderful tradtional dish found throughout the Americas in which the fish is "cooked" through the acids of citrus juices, such as lime, lemon, and orange) or grilled with a sprinkle of spice and fresh lemon juice. The American Heart Association (AHA) recommends eating fish at least two times a week, and Latin Americans have naturally been following AHA recommendations for years. My patients and viewers know that I've been touting the virtues of eating fish for a long time (hey, I come from an island!!).

Seriously, I've learned—and I share this with my patients, audience, and friends—that in addition to being a good source of protein without the high saturated fat found in many meat products, there are many additional health benefits to seafood. For example, because they're high in two kinds of omega-3 fatty acids, seafoods not only decrease the risk of arrhythmias that can lead to sudden cardiac death but also decrease blood clot formation that can lead to heart attacks and strokes, and lower the level of blood fats called triglycerides. These facts alone should push you right out the door to your favorite fishmonger! Another fish-related perk is that cooking it is simple. Peruvians—with their sashimi-like *tiradito*, which is essentially carpaccio of incredibly fresh fish—know that one of the secrets to eating fresh fish is pure elegance: dress it up lightly and the flavors—along with the healthy benefits—will shine. And there are so many varieties of easy-to-prepare and tasty white fish available in the States, like the Chilean congrio.

POULTRY IS PLUS

From luscious Colombian grilled quail with pepper sauce, to a Mexican pozole—chicken soup flavored with garlic, onion, cilantro, lime, and more—to allspice-, cinnamon-, and cayenne-sparked turkey prepared Caribbean style, Latin America offers a treasure trove of poultry recipes. Don't be afraid to use poultry in recipes that traditionally request meat; substituting ground turkey for ground beef in many dishes—like chilis and casseroles—reduces the amount of animal fats in the diet with just a slight difference in flavor. My advice when it comes to poultry? Enjoy what Latin Americans have been savoring for years: poultry with a dash of wildness! Poultry must be free-range, and preferably organic. Lean organic turkey and chicken are very good sources of high-density, low-fat protein produced without the added and potentially harmful chemicals. Organic poultry is a good source of selenium, zinc, niacin, vitamin E, beta-carotene, and vitamins B_6 and B_{12}. According to the USDA Sustainable Agriculture Research and Education Program, free-range organic poultry allowed access to the outdoors has 21 percent less total fat, 30 percent less saturated fat, 28 percent fewer calories, 50 percent more vitamin A, and 100 percent more omega-3 fatty acid than poultry not allowed outdoor access. And take that fatty skin off, please!

Don't forget about the egg! If you've lived in or visited Latin America, you've seen how many eggs are around; they've made their way atop many a garbanzo bean salad, or joined raisins, meat, and olives in an empanada. Though their cholesterol content once led to bad press, the American Heart Association has given eggs the go-ahead for healthy people. Eggs are full of high-quality protein and are the best sources of dietary choline, an essential nutrient (especially for pregnant women). Eggs have been shown to supply other nutrients that promote eye health and help prevent age-related macular degeneration, the leading cause of blindness in older people. As always, with any food, it's about variety and balance.

MORE ON MEAT

I wouldn't be honest if I told you, one, that meat is not part of the Latin American diet, and two, that I don't eat it! We're not talking Texas-style T-bones here; I'm talking the leaner cuts used for the fabulous Argentine *carne asadas* (fresh grilled low-fat cuts of beef cooked to perfection; can you hear me drooling?), or a Colombian *sobrebarriga*—flank steak—marinated in tomatoes, onion, garlic, and cumin and oven-cooked to fork tenderness. Lamb—one of the most hypoallergenic meats in the world—has been in the Americas for centuries thanks to the Europeans, but seasoned our way. It's our attitude about meat—and our incorporation of the deep flavors of spices, herbs, and vegetables—as well as a myriad of plant-based side dishes that make our approach to eating meat different. Latin Americans are a bit more discriminating in their approach to meat eating; it's not as extensive as it may be here in America.

SALSA

It's amazing how this lovely condiment has made a trailblazing trip up north, increasing momentum and its fan base as it goes. Essentially *salsa* is the Spanish word for sauce; using salsas as a condiment is a way of adding lots of flavor without adding a lot of fat. Take fresh mango salsa, for example, which can be made simply of fresh mango, red onion, fresh cucumber, and an optional diced jalapeño (I like a touch of spark!) with a splash of olive oil and white balsamic vinegar. You could add that to a piece of grilled chicken or fish—instead of a heftier and fattier dip or sauce—and have a zest of healthy flavors! Like herbs and spices, salsas can enhance and complement a main dish. And also like spices and herbs, there are so many wonderful combinations to explore.

SPICE IS LIFE

One of the things that makes this diet so healthful is its use of herbs (fresh whenever possible) and spices that complement the ingredients and add depth without the fat. This trick—the less fat and more flavor trick—has been traditionally practiced in Latin America for centuries. It's the technique of using sprinkles of cumin, oregano, and cilantro, which add not only taste but also health benefits. In fact, cumin, which is a great replacement for salt in many dishes, has been found to have ten times the antioxidant power of vitamin C. And it could also help protect against cancer. Parsley's cousin, cilantro, an herb included in many Latin American recipes, is said to contain antibiotic properties. And those red-hot chile peppers—not the group, mind you—don't just add plenty of spark to your dishes. There's something called capsaicin in hot peppers that offers a whole host of benefits: it helps digestion, fights against stomach ills like diarrhea, bacterial infections, and even heart disease. In fact, it's been associated with lowering blood pressure, reducing cholesterol, and even warding off strokes and heart attacks. And even beyond that, new research indicates that capsaicin actually reduces cancer cell growth in laboratory experiments. Well, it's not like I needed an excuse to have *my* food sparky, but now I'm giving you yours!

Now I don't want you to worry if many of these ingredients seem new or "foreign" to you. I promise that once you bring these into your life, you'll quickly be taken with their charm! And I also don't want you to worry if you think you can't find some of these ingredients; thanks to the Internet, it's easier than ever to find items that were previously only available south of the border. Most important, incorporating these key components into your daily diet should be simple—and tasty.

The Hot Latin Diet Versus Other Diets

Now that you know the fundamental foods behind the Latin diet, you need to find out what it will do for you. But first you need to make that decision: decide that it's time to move forward with a healthy and more fulfilling lifestyle. You need to make a commitment; you need to realize that changing your body for the better is going to require well-channeled passion—and effort. This, of course, is not easy. But I'm here for you—and I am promising to guide you along so that you feel both supported and educated by the process. In essence, the Hot Latin Diet is about building a way of life.

You may have tried a myriad of diets making similar promises. So you may ask yourself: What makes the Hot Latin Diet different from other diets? Well, let's take a look.

When I was in med school, many moons ago, there was one diet—hugely popular at the time—that caught my attention: the Scarsdale Diet. Do you remember this one? Developed by Dr. Herman Tarnower, this diet promised a one-pound-per-day weight loss. There was no calorie counting for this one, but food intake was strictly limited to specified amounts of fruits, vegetables, and mostly lean sources of protein. Artificial sweeteners and herbal appetite suppressants were often encouraged, while exercise was not. This diet was high in protein, low in carbohydrates, and moderate in fat, and required a seven-to-fourteen-day participation period, but then people were told to go off of it. Unfortunately, this left many poor souls with a very temporary weight-loss solution. After years of watching and studying the evolution of dieting, one fact is obvious: fad diets are fleeting. Also, there is an overwhelming number of diets out there. It seems like I'm interviewing nutritionists and diet gurus all the time about the latest claim to the best way to lose weight. Beyond that, my patients are constantly seeking dietary advice because they want to get back to their pre-pregnancy shape, or in some cases, just get healthier. When it comes to choosing a diet, the choices are overwhelming, and it can be difficult to determine which plan will yield the results you are looking for. All diets are going to promise you weight loss. The fact of the matter is, if you put any overweight person on a regimen, she will lose weight quickly. So what makes one better than the other? I'm now going to go through some of the popular (and not-so-popular) diets to give you the scoop, and highlight the important factors you should look for in any diet. As you may know, many diets, as in several mentioned here, were initially developed by physicians for their patients. It's important to note that these diets were created with their innovator's best intentions; the doctors used their expertise to develop what they believed were healthful and effective weight loss plans.

THE ATKINS STORY

You've most likely heard of this diet because it remains one of the most controversial fad diets around. Developed by the late Dr. Robert C. Atkins, this diet is best known for its carbohydrate-restricting rules. This very rigid program allows practically no carbohydrates, especially during the beginning stages, while encouraging large amounts of protein. As a result of consuming practically no carbohydrates, the dieter's body goes into something called ketosis, a state in which the body begins to burn off its stores of fat because it thinks that it's being starved. As a result, the initial weight loss is usually pretty quick, but the sudden drop in carbohydrates can produce a variety of side effects, ranging from dizziness to bad breath.

There are a lot of saturated fat–rich foods allowed on this diet, so people who are into their cheese, butter, cream, bacon, and so on, enjoy having free range in that area. This diet—packed with fat and low in carbs—has many health-conscious folks worried for several reasons. Perhaps the most important is that the long-term effects are still unknown.

What I like

▶ This diet leads to rapid weight loss.

▶ This diet permits dieters to eat unlimited protein-rich and fatty foods.

▶ This diet is not as time-consuming nor as expensive as some of the other popular diets.

What I don't like

▶ It's very restrictive.

▶ It supports the high consumption of saturated fats.

▶ It can cause bad breath, nausea, and headaches (especially in the beginning phase).

▶ This diet relies heavily upon proteins from meat, fish, and dairy products, so it wouldn't work for vegetarians. Also, by default, it cuts out many valuable nutrients. Furthermore, there are concerns about the effect of such high levels of protein and fat upon vital organs, such as the heart and kidneys.

ENTER THE SOUTH BEACH DIET

The South Beach Diet, developed by the cardiologist Arthur Agatston, is based on the conclusion that Americans are crazy for carbohydrates. In fact, the two-week induction phase of virtually no carbs is designed to help people stop craving them, and they're subsequently minimized throughout the diet. In the first two weeks of this diet, bread, cereal, fruit, potatoes, rice, pasta, beets, carrots, and corn are not allowed. (Even after that, most of these foods remain strongly discouraged.) Absolutely no beer, wine, or other alcohol is permitted during the first fourteen days.

The reason for this is that according to the South Beach theory, highly processed carbohydrates are digested too quickly, which makes insulin levels (a hormone the body makes to process sugars) spike. When these carbs are used up, your elevated insulin level makes you desire more food—especially carbohydrates. The South Beach Diet's goal is to break this cycle of eating and wanting carbs, and to make you want to eat less—and better—food.

Actually, in both the South Beach and Atkins diets, there are severe induction phases, followed by long-term eating plans. The differences between the two lie in two areas: fats and carbs. The South Beach Diet prohibits unhealthy fats but strongly encourages healthy ones. Also, the South Beach Diet doesn't count grams of carbohydrates. The South Beach Diet looks at how much sugar is in a carb. Low-sugar carbs—those with a low glycemic index (they don't cause the blood-sugar levels to rise and fall as quickly)—are good.

What I like

▶ This diet is pretty balanced after the initial highly regimented phase.

▶ This diet does not rely on high levels of saturated fat.

▶ This diet doesn't require calorie or fat counting.

▶ This diet encourages regular meals and snacking.

What I don't like

▶ It's quite difficult for people who are used to high-carb diets.

▶ This diet can be costly in terms of time and money.

▶ This diet is not for life—so many people go back into their old eating habits, and thus gain the pounds right back.

THE ZONE

Developed by Barry Sears, Ph.D., a former researcher in biotechnology at the Massachusetts Institute of Technology, the Zone professes that a diet high in carbohydrates and low in protein and fats is unhealthy. Essentially Sears's thinking is that the body functions at its ideal metabolic rate if each of us consumes the right amount of protein, fats, and carbohydrates (30 percent, 30 percent, and 40 percent, respectively). This ratio applies to all meals all the time. While this diet does not recommend that you eat fewer calories than you're currently consuming, it suggests you eat different ones—and that you're careful about your portions. In his book, Sears gives you a list of foods allowed both at mealtime and for snacks. There are a wide range of foods allowed and no confusing schedules or conditions that need to be memorized. Though dieters may find it easy to follow, nutritionists have given this diet mixed reviews. Numerous health experts argue that there are much safer and better diets than the Zone diet. They say that the Five a Day system, which encourages people to eat five servings of fruits and vegetables a day, is much more nutritionally sound. The American Heart Association has even issued an official recommendation warning against diets like the Zone stating that most of these diets do not provide a balanced level of nutrients that our bodies need. Furthermore, though many have reported rapid weight loss from the Zone diet, they've also, consequently, reported a subsequent rapid weight gain.

What I like

▶ This diet can help with rapid weight loss.

▶ This diet educates people in both portion control and sugar reduction.

▶ This is a vegetable- and fruit-rich diet.

▶ Dieters say that after a few days their cravings for processed carbs begin to disappear.

What I don't like

▶ Though rapid weight loss is listed as an advantage, many dieters know that this is quickly and frequently followed by rapid weight gain.

▶ This diet is not practical for many people.

▶ This diet can be expensive to follow.

▶ This diet restricts some valuable vitamins and minerals.

▶ This diet can be very time-consuming and anxiety-producing because you have to measure everything.

THE SUGAR BUSTERS DIET

Quite similar to the Zone diet is the Sugar Busters diet, which was developed in the 1990s by a group of medical professionals: Samuel S. Andrews, M.D., Morrison C. Bethea, M.D., Luis A. Balart, M.D., and H. Leighton Steward, MSc and the CEO of a Fortune 500 energy company. The Sugar Busters diet—like the Zone diet—recommends that daily calorie intake is split into a 40/30/30 ratio; however, the percentage distributions are different. In the Zone diet, the higher 40 percent ratio is made up of carbohydrates; the Sugar Busters diet recommends that 40 percent of daily calorie intake be made up of fat, that 30 percent be made up of protein, and that the final 30 percent be made up of carbohydrates.

What I like

▶ The diet cuts out many foods that are clearly unhealthy, including refined sugar.

▶ There is no calorie counting on this diet.

▶ This diet encourages exercise.

What I don't like

▶ This diet cuts out some valuable minerals and nutrients.

▶ This diet does not work for vegetarians.

▶ Weight loss is probably due to the calorie reduction, not the 40/30/30 ratio.

▶ This diet restricts some fruits and vegetables.

WEIGHT WATCHERS

Since the early 1960s, Weight Watchers, which began when a few friends started meeting weekly to discuss how to best lose weight, has taught people how to plan a more balanced diet, control cravings and impulses, and increase physical activity. Weight Watchers offers dieters the added bonus of group support, through either weekly meetings or online communities. According to this diet, foods and exercise are calculated into a point plan, which essentially translates into an education and the practice of eating better foods and moving your body more.

What I like

▶ Support is offered to people on this diet.

▶ This diet does not exclude major food groups.

▶ Vegetarians can participate in this diet plan.

▶ This diet makes it easier than others to eat outside the home.

What I don't like

▶ The portion control doesn't educate people about amounts they should be eating once they're off the diet (since everything on the diet is premeasured for them).

▶ The point system doesn't always indicate the nutritional value of foods.

▶ The prepackaged foods leave you with less choices, less healthy alternatives, and without an education of what you could eat on your own.

▶ This diet can be costly in terms of both time and money.

THE 3-HOUR DIET

Jorge Cruise's shtick is timing. His diet—the 3-Hour Diet—is not so much based on what you eat but when and how much you eat. He advocates eating breakfast within one hour of rising, and then eating every three hours thereafter—but stopping three hours before bedtime. Cruise says that eating this way increases BMR (baseline metabolic rate, which indicates how fast your body burns calories) and energy, while it decreases your appetite. In terms of what you eat, Cruise believes there are no bad foods, just bad portions. He says that meals should be about 400 calories each, and that learning to eat the right portion, at the right time, will yield success. However, while people do report successful weight loss on this plan, it's not clear as to whether it's a metabolic improvement as a result of spreading three meals out into five or six smaller meals.

What I like

▶ This diet recognizes the importance of frequent eating.

▶ It also recognizes portion and caloric control.

What I don't like

▶ It is expected that this diet will work without requiring any increase in exercise.

▶ This diet includes processed snacks that are virtually void of nutritional value (like Reese's Peanut Butter Cups and Chips Ahoy!).

CABBAGE SOUP AND LEMONADE

There are so many of these quick-fix diets out there, and they have all kinds of gimmicks. They frequently require a lot of prep time, which may not always be practical. While these diets can be very seductive as far as promises for rapid weight loss, I urge you to think about the fact they are not healthy and, in fact, can have negative consequences. Here's a snapshot of a couple of them.

The Cabbage Soup Diet promises quick results after consuming strange and bizarre combinations of a super-strict regimen of food for seven days. This plan, like many others of its kind, is certainly not nutritionally sound and is certainly not one for a lifetime! Any diet that requires you to consume a single food for several days in a row is not a healthy one. The Lemonade—or Master Cleanse Diet—also falls into this category.

Developed by the late naturopath Stanley Burroughs, the Master Cleanse Diet consists of fasting to rid the body of toxins. The idea is that a special lemonade—made with maple syrup and cayenne pepper—will clean you out and get rid of harmful toxins while promising weight loss of about two pounds a day for most people. Like other fad diets, detox regimens promise quick weight losses that are—at the end of the day—unsustainable. Based on popular thinking, as opposed to educated research, extreme diets like the Master Cleanse can cause serious side effects in vulnerable groups.

Whether you're looking at Atkins or Dr. Phil—and all the ones that crop up in between—most diets are nothing more than low-calorie nutrition plans glossed up through skillful marketing gimmicks. In fact, fad diets are very easy to identify: they usually either push or prohibit a particular food. And their advice is certainly not in line with recognized experts and organizations, like the American Dietetic Association and the American Heart Association. Fad diets can provide an unhealthy quick fix. What they do is significantly slow down your metabolism—and then, when you're off the diet, your body is slow to regain its previous metabolic speed (which obviously contributes to your already big chances of gaining weight back). Also, because they typically restrict major nutrients, they can lead to serious health problems later on; this is exactly what we're *not* looking for. For example, let's say you go on a fad diet that limits your caloric intake to 1,000 calories a day for a month. Your body has an instinctual response to adjust. Though at first you will drop a few pounds, if you continue with this significant drop in calories, after even less than a week the body will say, "Okay, we're having a famine. We need to make adjustments." So what happens is it begins to preserve nutrients in order to "protect" you. You stop losing weight, and your metabolism slows down to accommodate the lesser amount of fuel it's receiving.

Just to recap—there are a few more warnings about fad diets that I'd like to give you:

▶ Diets that restrict eating to one or two foods are not nutritionally sound and can even be dangerous over time (not to mention boring and difficult to follow).

▶ When supplements or special supplements are part of a diet, you could end up shelling out a great deal of cash. This money would be much better spent stocking your fridge and pantry with healthy—and delicious—choices.

▶ Weight loss through fad diets is often temporary and short term; in fact, many dieters report gaining back all the weight lost—and more!

▶ Exercise—as I've said before—must be part of your daily routine to help you tone your body, boost your immune system, elevate your moods, and increase your energy.

Why the Hot Latin Diet?

With all these diet touters out there, you might ask why I am here doing the same thing. The answer, my friend, is simple: I'm not doing the same thing. The Hot Latin Diet has the best approach to weight loss by offering realistic goals that apply specifically to your needs, practical solutions, and long-lasting effects. This diet focuses on the most important and fundamental lessons of nutrition and teaches you how to make smart choices when it comes to food. Restrictions are on fat but never on taste; the seven Latin powerfoods integral to this diet are not only full of vital nutrients, antioxidants, and even medicinal properties but are also fresh and organic, delicious, and easy to prepare. Not only will I reveal the untapped secrets of these foods, but I will also show you which food combinations provide the most optimal health benefits and promote fast weight loss. Also, there is an assortment of lean meats and seafood, vegetables, fruits, nuts, and whole grains, making food preparation fun and flexible! You'll never get bored when you follow this diet.

Along with providing you with the most optimal foods, this diet also teaches you how to shed pounds and maintain your desired weight without having to obsessively count calories. Your metabolism will become more efficient through portion control, smaller but more frequent meals, and smart snacking.

Finally, the results from this diet don't stop once you reach your goal. The most fundamental guidelines on food, nutrition, exercise, and stress management are listed to teach you how to maintain your weight. It's realistic that life can get in the way of any plan, so it is important to be prepared and flexible. That's why this diet also offers simple and practical solutions for when you gain some of the weight back, or if you find yourself steering off track. This philosophy is the basis of the Hot Latin Diet, the reward of which is a healthy and happy lifestyle.

Making the Hot Latin Diet Work for You

You have to make this diet work for *you*. Make it fit your lifestyle and the needs of your age group. Below you will find brief descriptions regarding the specific needs of each age group. These tips and guidelines will help you execute this plan as effectively as possible.

THE TWENTIES AND THIRTIES

At this point, many of you are on your way to careers but you may not have started a family yet. Because you feel so energetic (hopefully!), you may not be as concerned about diet as you should be. But even if you're young and thin and going to the gym regularly, you still need to be careful about what you're eating.

As I wrote in *The Checklist*, it seems like Americans pay more attention to the gas they put in their cars than the food they put in their mouths! As kids, many of us might learn about nutrition—if we're paying attention—in health classes. But beyond that, unless your parents were into it, you're probably not too well versed in nutrition. Unfortunately, our lack of knowledge, combined with our obsession with processed foods, is really damaging our health. What we really need to do is what the Hot Latin Diet does: get back to fundamentals. Eating a diet that is well balanced, with vegetables and fruit, fish and lean meat, and good unsaturated fats like olive oil will help (see page 3—the list of my seven Latin powerfoods).

But it's not just *what* or *how much* you're eating; it's *the way* you're eating. That's why I say that in your twenties or thirties, if you haven't been eating correctly, you need to change that! Well, no time like the present.

Many of you are probably doing the out-the-door-without-eating thing: you simply get up and go. And your lunchtime habits may not be any better. So let's say you skip breakfast, gulp down a midday lunch, and then eat a large dinner at around seven or so. The problem is, when you're in your twenties or thirties, you don't need all that fuel at night; you need a little throughout the day if you're active—moving, thinking, or both. Actually, there are consequences to eating like this: without a supply of energy, your metabolism gets altered. Your blood sugar is erratic and your hormones go crazy trying to figure out where to get the fuel they need.

Ideally, for optimal energy consumption and metabolism, you should eat small meals every three hours. (Check out my recipes on pages 95–153!) So if you eat breakfast at seven o'clock in the morning, you could have a snack at ten, lunch at one, a snack at four, and dinner at about seven. And don't forget to drink plenty of water (preferably not tap, but filtered or spring), which is essential for cellular metabolism, in between! This way of eating will translate into an effective burning of fuel—and a high energy level—all day long.

THE FORTIES AND FIFTIES

If you're here, then you know the deal: without warning, your oh-so-efficient metabolism starts to slow down and the pounds start to add up. Suddenly your slim waistline starts to grow wider—and now everything looks and feels tighter and unflattering. It's frustrating, to say the least!

Being menopausal—or perimenopausal—certainly doesn't help! The good news is that there are so many things you can do to better adapt to menopause, and diet and exercise are key helpers. In fact, many physicians believe that many of the symptoms of menopause can be traced to a poor diet (as well as an unhealthy lifestyle and environmental pollutants).

But let's talk about menopause and diet, which play a huge role in our metabolism. A healthy diet is more important now than before because your risks of osteoporosis (extreme bone loss) and heart disease go up at this stage of life. A diet rich in whole grains, leafy greens, and other fruits and vegetables is essential for normal hormone production. Add calcium-rich foods (leafy green vegetables, nuts and seeds, and seafood, as well as organic natural dairy) or take a calcium supplement to obtain your recommended daily intake (see page 78). Get adequate vitamin D from sunshine or a supplement. Avoid alcohol and caffeine, which can also trigger hot flashes in some women. And of course, follow the tips and recipes in *The Hot Latin Diet*, as well as moving and shaking that body (check out my section on exercising starting on page 177). If you're doing the opposite—eating fast foods and trans-fatty acids (man-made processed fats and oils)—then you're not getting the antioxidants, vitamins, and minerals you need to neutralize the effects of both the harmful environmental hormones you're exposed to and the harmful by-products of your own metabolism. This will, in turn, not only exacerbate your mood swings but increase your waistline—and more—even more!

THE SIXTIES AND BEYOND

The good news is that if you've taken good care of yourself, you'll now reap the benefits. The better news is that it's never too late to start being healthy! This is the time when you should watch your weight, lessen your consumption of saturated fat, and become even more physically active. As always, choose from the list of seven Latin powerfoods whenever possible; you need foods rich in calcium, as well as nutrient-dense foods like fish, poultry, lean meat, low-fat dairy products, fruits and vegetables, whole-grain cereals, nuts, and seeds.

Also, you should eat more frequently; five to six small, low-fat meals daily may help to control weight, blood-fat levels, and blood sugar. Make sure you're drinking enough water, because as you age your need for fluids gets even greater. Sip fluids—primarily water (or nonsugary beverages)—throughout the day.

How to Execute the Plan

By this point, you know what the benefits of the seven Latin power-foods and their subcategories are, you understand the fundamentals of this diet and how it compares to others you may have tried or heard of, and you know how to tailor the diet to your age category. Now the question is how to execute the plan. The answer is through three simple tracks.

TRACK ONE (FIRST TWO WEEKS)

Once you decide to make this lifestyle change, you will feel it. The first two weeks include a variety of recipes that are probably low(er) in fat and calories than what you normally consume, as well as nutritionally well-rounded dishes. There are several seafood and fish dishes, which contain proteins that are easier to digest than red meat options (they're also adaptable). Also, the recipes include more raw fruits and vegetables, which have a higher water content and will help flush out toxins. You should feel energetic and strong, as well as acutely aware of the benefits of your new way of life. You might not have those sluggish moments you had from either a lack of eating or eating the wrong foods.

TRACK TWO (NEXT FOUR WEEKS)

Thanks to the fact that your cells are enjoying "high-octane fuel" and you're eradicating toxins, you're starting to see more significant changes in your body and in your energy levels. You will need to keep up your high standards for nutrition, but now you can start to incorporate some richer ingredients for maintenance of strength, muscle mass, power, and stamina. You should incorporate the recipes you've been enjoying from Track One along with the new ones.

Basically, at this point your body is working in synch with the high quality of foods you're providing it, and that, along with your increased movement, is helping you to "spring clean" areas of your body, sending signals that fat deposits can be metabolized, which leads to effective weight loss. Furthermore, you're building areas that need it: your weak bones are becoming stronger, as is your muscle mass (which is the key fat burner). Not only are you getting rid of fat, your body is working thanks to your ingesting of complex carbs, good fat, and good protein. By the end of Track Two, you can expect to have decreased your body fat by 8 percent to 10 percent and to have lost about twelve to eighteen pounds.

TRACK THREE (WEEK SEVEN AND BEYOND)

This is the time when your new habits have become an integrated part of your lifestyle. You've learned about the benefits of good foods, portion control, and physical activity. You also realize that quick fixes are not the answer, but that gradual, enduring life changes are. Enjoy continuing to mix and match the recipes from all the tracks. You're also able to forgive yourself for mistakes that you make; we are, after all, human! Through these three simple and fun-to-follow tracks, you will achieve your weight-loss goals while preserving your figure and living a life full of flavor, zest, and happiness.

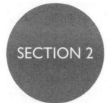

SECTION 2

GETTING STARTED AND SETTING YOUR GOALS

☑ *Setting Up Your Everyday Life for Success*

☑ *Reading Food Labels*

☑ *Setting Your Goals*

☑ *Your Goals*

Setting Up Your Everyday Life for Success

In order to truly lose weight and stay healthy, you need to revamp the world around you. The two areas in your life that you need to change immediately are your closet and your kitchen.

THE CLOSET

Since we've talked a lot about approach, now is the time to get down to the nitty-gritty. If you're like many women I've spoken with, you have that one untouched dress you'll wear when you've lost some weight; it's the dress that you know will make you look and feel just gorgeous—when, of course, the time is right. You bought it as an incentive . . . but you're not at the point when you can wear it. And, in fact, when you got discouraged, you hung it right behind those hide-everything black pants. Well, my friend, pull that baby out. It's time to tackle the big C: your closet.

As I've mentioned before, part of getting ready to diet is the visualization of your goal. This is the more proactive part about getting ready—and, like everything else that promises rewards, it's tough! But it's part of a very important process in this whole diet thing. So here are my top seven closet-cleaning suggestions:

1. Put aside a block of time on a day that doesn't have you otherwise occupied with work, family, or other obligations (but procrastinators, this doesn't mean next month!), and decide that you're going to spend a two-to-three-hour chunk of time (and maybe more) on this project.

2. Bring some of those big black garbage bags—and a storage box—with you.

3. Put on your favorite tunes, get yourself something to sip on (no cocktails yet!), put on your cleaning clothes, and let's get started.

4. Set up certain stations in your bedroom for dresses, pants, shirts, skirts, shoes, and so on. Now take out everything. I know this is a huge mess, but this is part of the process. (And unless you want to keep some dust bunnies as pets, this is a perfect opportunity to clean—and to give yourself a bit of exercise in addition to a clean closet!)

5. Start with one pile at a time, and make sub-piles according to the following categories:

   - Giveaway pile (If you haven't worn it for twelve months or just don't like it anymore, it's time to say good-bye.)

   - What-fits-me-now pile

   - When-I'm-thinner pile

   - And finally, the out-of-season pile

(Though I'm not addressing the shoes here, I strongly suggest the same giveaway policy.)

6. Take the one outfit from the when-I'm-thinner pile that you'd most like to wear and put that to one aside. Place the giveaway pile in one of those bags (to be carted off later to the donation of your choice), and the items from the out-of-season pile into a box for storage until the season's right.

7. Take that when-I'm-thinner garment, clean and press it, and then hang it in an easy-to-reach location. This piece, which will work even better than your scale, will reward you when you've achieved your goal!

Now you should have a big bag of giveaway clothes, and hopefully a more modest pile of keepers, which you can now—according to color or article—hang up in your newly cleaned closet. Oh, and don't forget to do the same for those clothes in drawers, though you may want to hold off at least until another day (but don't wait too long)! Now that you've cleaned out the closet and drawers, you should feel good; you've taken a fundamental step in the right direction and you're ready to continue. Realize, of course, that one of the nicest parts of losing weight—aside from feeling great, looking hot, and being healthier—is that you can fit into clothes that you couldn't work with before.

We all know that clothes can be pretty pricey, but they can also be a wonderful incentive. When you hit your target weight, buy yourself a beautiful—and, yes, expensive—outfit. This is not only to acquire a gorgeous piece of clothing that helps you show off that new hot figure of yours, it's also a kind of insurance. Think of it this way: When you invest in a new car, you do your best to keep it clean, right? You make sure it stays as pristine and undented as possible; you put a lot of attention into keeping that car looking good and running well. The same could be said when you spend a lot of your hard-earned cash on a new outfit; you're going to make sure you take good care of yourself—and of it—so that you get your money's worth! This is one way to reward yourself *and* to keep your inspiration going.

THE KITCHEN

Now it's time to start on the next big area of change: the kitchen. Cleaning out your food sources in the kitchen serves three big purposes. First, you'll get rid of those temptations that can sometimes sabotage your best efforts. That seductive bag of chips, or creamy all-sugar, all-fat peanut butter, or the "kids'" candy that you can't resist would be best left out of your home altogether! Why torture yourself, especially when you're just getting started! Second, you'll be able to do a kind of inventory, and recognize some of your soon-to-be-outdated eating habits. Third, you'll be left with a clean and well-organized fridge and pantry! This will help set up a clean slate for you, and increase your chances of success. Actually, when you think about it, your body is like your kitchen: both should be filled with healthy foods. Also, make sure you have measuring cups (and spoons!) in your kitchen. These will not only help you with the recipes, they'll also help you with another key component of the Hot Latin Diet: portion control.

FRIDGE FIRST

Cleaning out your fridge—and your pantry—can be a cathartic exercise for many reasons. First, you're removing foods, condiments, snacks—temptations—that are much more easily avoided if invisible (out of sight, out of mind!). But even better than that, you're clarifying for yourself what you should and shouldn't ingest. So when you have those pieces of pizza in your fridge left over from last night's supper, the best thing to do, my friend, is to get rid of the temptation. Otherwise, I know that you'll want to eat them.

WHAT SHOULD YOU GET RID OF?

Before you start cleaning, grab yourself a pad and pen. As you're on your fridge dig, note what you find—and how many calories each represents. (If you've got your computer nearby, you can tally it all up on www.calorie-count.com/.) And now on to the fridge dig:

I can't speak for everyone in this country, but if your refrigerator looks anything like mine did before I started the Hot Latin Diet, I might be able to guess which typical high-fat foods lurk in the corners. There are certain foods—comfort foods, if you will—that have an emotional hold on us, making us believe that we can't live without them. But if you take a look at the calories, it might make you think twice about your priorities. Here are the foods I eventually had to ban from my refrigerator; if even some of these items sound familiar, just know that you are in good company: mac and cheese (about 600 calories); Chinese fried rice or takeout (about 720); chocolate cake with frosting (fab stuff—but a whopping 853 calories in one piece!); roast beef hero (500 calories); lasagna (1,020 calories); a selection of cold cuts (about 300 calories, though lean meat such as turkey is fine); hot dogs (still good, still unopened, but so much salt . . . and 350 calories for one with a roll); cheese, which I love almost as much as chocolate cake (about 1,000 calories); lemonade from concentrate (200 calories); and a couple of cans of soda (184 calories). Now on to the condiments: mayo (90 calories per tablespoon), and many more of your favorite toppings, including sugar-laden vinaigrettes and salad dressings (about 500 calories).

If you do the math, that adds up to more than 6,000 calories! Imagine how much different you and your life would be just by eliminating these foods. So let's begin by going down a typical list of what to remove from your fridge and what to keep.

What to Remove from Your Fridge

hot dogs

processed cheese

processed foods

processed lunch meats

soft drinks

packaged dessert items

sugar-sweetened yogurt

processed and bottled salad dressings

condiments like ketchup and mayonnaise

margarine

high-fat cuts of meat (i.e., any cut that has
visible white fat or that is marbled).

jellies and jams (or use very little!)

What to Keep in Your Fridge

low-fat dairy or soy products

fresh eggs

fresh vegetables like tomatillos and
avocados (Latin powerfoods!)

fresh whole fruit (like limes and lemons
for seasoning)

fresh greens

fresh chiles (one of the seven Latin
powerfoods!)

lean meats and poultry

fish fillets, steaks, or chunks of tuna
or salmon

low-sodium soy sauce

cilantro (a Latin powerfood!) and other
fresh herbs for seasoning

a variety of
nuts and nut butters (but don't overdo
the nut butters; check the serving
size—between 1 and 2 tablespoons—
and stick to it!)

What to Remove from Your Freezer

ice cream

frozen fries

frozen high-fat prepared foods

What to Put in Your Freezer

frozen fruits

frozen juice bars with no sugar added

frozen vegetables that have no added
ingredients (check the label!)

PANTRY NEXT

The refrigerator is not the only food space that needs to be reevaluated. In fact, many, if not all, dry, processed foods that are stored in pantries are even worse for your health and diet, as they tend to be high in sugar and preservatives. Sugar-laden cereals, chips, candy, flavor-enhanced seasonings, soups, and canned fruits—all these foods are definite red flags and should be disposed of immediately if you want to get on the track to healthy living.

The pantry is also the home of many spices. Something you may not be aware of is that in order to make the most of your seasoning, you should replace your spices every six months. Most herbs and spices contain oils that evaporate during storage, which reduces their flavor and strength. If you consider the fact that the spices and herbs you find in the supermarket have probably been sitting on the shelves for a while (and probably in a warehouse before then), you can see they've already aged considerably. If you can buy your spices and herbs from a fresher source, that's best. Besides, it's not only fresher, it's usually

What to Remove from Your Pantry	*What to Keep in Your Pantry*
white bread	whole-grain bread
breakfast cereals that are not sugar coated, but are not whole grain either	whole-grain cereals
	whole-grain pasta
meat snacks, like beef jerky, that have a lot of additives	healthy snack bars
dry mixes, like macaroni and cheese	olive, or grapeseed, flaxseed, sesame, walnut, and peanut oils **Note:** *(They're all from plants, and are a healthy way to replace the unhealthy fats in your diet, but must be used in moderation.)*
boxed dinner mixes	
pasta and noodles and tortillas made from regular white flour	

cheaper if you can find a bulk retailer. Now, let's start tidying up that pantry using the list below as a guide.

REFILLING THOSE SHELVES

Now that you've done the big clean, it's time to restock. Review the list I've given you above, as well as the shopping list below. Also, I want you to keep something in mind: Buy what you need and don't keep unhealthy foods on hand (this will only lead to temptation, which, as you well know, can avalanche). Also, if you have a family, don't be suckered into refilling with junk; remember that you can all benefit by having healthy snacks around.

Shopping List

ají amarillo (jarred Peruvian yellow pepper, available in Latin markets and large supermarkets)

almond extract

black beans (canned or dried)

black pepper

brown sugar (dark)

canola oil

cayenne pepper

chickpeas (canned or dried)

chile de árbol powder

chili powder

chipotle en adobo (in cans)

cinnamon

coarse and/or kosher salt

corn tortilla chips

cumin seeds

dark balsamic vinegar

dark brown sugar

dark rum

Dijon mustard

evaporated skim milk

extra-virgin olive oil

fava beans

fennel seeds

ground cumin

ground ginger

habanero powder

huitlacoche (also called cuitlacoche; a Mexican specialty, available in cans in some Latin markets)

kosher salt

(continued)

Shopping List (continued)

light coconut milk

Mexican oregano

mirin (Japanese rice cooking wine)

olive oil

organic chicken broth

panko (Japanese-style bread crumbs)

peanut oil

pine nuts

porcini mushrooms (dried)

raw pumpkin seeds

red wine vinegar

sherry vinegar

sherry wine

shredded coconut (sweetened or unsweetened)

soursop (guanabana) nectar (Note: use sparingly or as indicated due to the high sugar content)

soy sauce (low sodium)

star anise

tahini paste

tomato paste

turbinado sugar

vanilla extract

vegetable oil

white balsamic vinegar

white wine

Reading Food Labels

Now that you're off to the supermarket to restock that kitchen, setting yourself up for success, let's take a quick lesson on reading food labels.

One of the most important steps in changing your lifestyle is monitoring yourself. Reading food labels will help you determine the kinds of food you're ingesting and, in some cases, whether or not you should be choosing a particular product.

First of all, when reading a label, make sure to notice the serving size. Many packaged foods will be advertised on the container as healthy and low-calorie or low-fat, but their serving sizes are tiny, so that they look like they have a low fat and sugar content.

This label, for example, gives you the nutritional information for carrots, and the serving size is 3 ounces, but there are 2½ servings in a

Nutrition Facts

Serving Size 1 Cup (85g) (3 oz.)
Servings Per Container 2.5

Amount Per Serving

Calories 45	Calories from Fat 0

	% Daily Value*
Total Fat 0g	0%
Saturated Fat 0g	0%
Cholesterol 0mg	0%
Sodium 55mg	2%
Total Carbohydrate 10g	3%
Dietary Fiber 3g	12%
Sugars 5g	
Protein 1g	

Vitamin A 360%	•	Vitamin C 8%
Calcium 2%	•	Iron 0%

*Percent Daily Values are based on a 2,000 calorie diet. Your daily value may be higher or lower depending on your calorie needs.

	Calories:	2,000	2,500
Total Fat	Less than	65g	80g
Sat. Fat	Less than	20g	25g
Cholesterol	Less than	300mg	300mg
Sodium	Less than	2,400mg	2,400mg
Total Carbohydrate	Less than	300mg	375mg
Dietary Fiber	Less than	25g	30g

Calories pergram: Fat 9 ▪ Carbohydrate 4 ▪ Protein 4   Ingredients: Carrots.

bag. You will need to take this into account when planning how much to eat at a meal or as a snack.

Next, the label tells you that there are 45 calories per serving. Just be sure to multiply the number of calories by the number of servings you plan to eat.

The calories from fat has to do with how many fat grams a food actually contains—and remember that each gram of fat adds up to 9 calories. In the case of carrots there are none, but in other foods you may notice that the fat calories are quite high in comparison to the total calories present in the food, like in the case of nuts, which contain 50 percent fat calories. In other words, let's say a serving of almond butter is 2 tablespoons, or 32 grams. The total calories is 195, out of which 150 are fat calories; this means that if each fat gram contains 9 calories, then half the grams of the almond butter serving is made of fat (that is because when you divide 150 calories by 9 calories you get approximately 16 grams). Then again, almond butter contains healthy fat, and I do not tell you to avoid healthy fat, just factor in how much is best for you to consume each day according to my guidelines in the daily servings chart.

Protein and carbohydrates contain 4 calories per gram. In the case of the carrots on this food label, which have 45 calories per serving, 41 calories are from carbohydrate, and 4 calories are from protein. Fiber does not contain calories, so the more fiber a food has, the better, since the fiber actually helps slow down the carbohydrate absorption in the body for better fuel usage.

The carbohydrate section of the label is divided into dietary fiber and sugars. Sugars are a very important section to look at. Do your best to avoid foods that have zero dietary fiber and more than 20 grams of sugars per serving, as most likely these are foods high in processed sugar that will spike your blood-sugar levels. Complex carbohydrates, such as tubers and whole grains, may be high in total carbohydrate content, but you will find that they have fiber in them and not such high sugar content. Foods high in fiber are the ones with 5 or more grams of fiber per serving.

Protein is protein, so there is not much to break down here, but do know that a food that contains some protein, fiber, and fat as well as carbohydrate, can go a long way to reduce the amount of sugar spiking in the bloodstream versus a food that is all carbohydrate without fiber, protein, or fat (such as white flour and white bread or sugar). Back to the fat section of the label: this is broken down into total fat as well as a subsection called saturated fat. Some labels will also list trans fats, and mono- and unsaturated fats. Avoid the ones with any grams of trans fats, and minimize the saturated fat grams. Mono- and unsaturated fats are the healthy fats, which I do recommend eating daily.

An important note: Processed foods often carry misleading food labels that hide important information. For instance, if you find a label that lists the total fat as, say, 20 grams per serving, and then the saturated and other fats do not add up to 20 grams total, then there are some grams of hydrogenated and trans fats in there that are not overtly listed. Tricky! These labels will not have the subsection "trans fats" listed on them. This is where you must thoroughly read the list of ingredients, which is given below the nutritional breakdown.

The ingredients are listed in order of content; the highest amount of an ingredient present is listed first. Again, you should examine this list carefully. A front label may announce a fruit juice that claims to be healthy, such as pure grape juice, but then, when you read the label, you could find the list of ingredients in this order: water, high-fructose corn syrup, apple juice from concentrate, grape juice from concentrate, flavorings. As you can see in this example, grape juice is near the end of the list.

Also, any foods that contain ingredients that are hard to pronounce and sound like man-made chemicals are best to avoid, such as partially hydrogenated vegetable oil, and monosodium glutamate (msg), and too many more to list here. Remember that dairy can be present in a food in the form of whey, and a sugar derived from dairy is called lactose. Also, sugar is present in many forms: sucrose, fructose, dextrose, high-fructose corn syrup, and maltose, among others. Also, artificial sweeteners include saccharin, xylitol, sugar alcohols, and many others. The best sugar to eat is the one naturally present in fresh fruit with nothing on it, and this is better than juice, which excludes the fiber present in the fruit.

The right-hand column lists the percentages of daily values per component of the food according to the amount of calories you eat in a day. In the case of most labels, they use 2,000 or 2,500 calories a day as a recommended daily allowance standard. So each food will list what percentage of carbohydrates, proteins, and fats are present per serving based on the total allowed each day. The same is done for the recommended amount of vitamins to be consumed each day, and what vitamins and minerals are present in that particular food.

As you're reading a label, please keep my suggestions in mind. It's best to eat as much unpackaged, fresh whole food as you can.

Setting Your Goals

Now that you're ready to get started, let's work on the first step to any diet—establishing your goals. The only way to truly set realistic and educated goals is to understand three key elements to dieting: weight gain, food and nutrition, and your body. After all, you are what you eat, and attaining this knowledge will help you make better choices when it comes to nutrition and food.

UNDERSTANDING THE TRUTH BEHIND WEIGHT GAIN

First, I have a confession: I used to never care about what I ate. Not only that, I also loved take-out foods—mostly because of my crazy work schedule. And oh, I wasn't the most athletic guy. In fact, I didn't start exercising until I was in my thirties, when suddenly I realized that I had to do something to keep my body healthy.

Does this sound familiar? Honestly, it seems like we've all got some pounds we could shed—and we're in big company (yes, pun intended). But seriously, this is no joking matter: the statistics about obesity in this country are far from funny. Can you believe that by 2010, three-quarters of the U.S. population will be overweight? And if that didn't shock you, check this out: statistics show that 80 percent of our kids are *currently* overweight. Did you also know that these kids are suffering from weight-related afflictions, like arthritis? The consequences of extra weight are devastating. So here's my question: how did we get here?

The Top Eight Factors That Contribute to Weight Gain

✔ FAST FOOD

Just one walk through a supermarket or down Main Street will explain part of the weight gain: our diets. You'd be hard-pressed to *not* find a plethora of fast foods in virtually every town in our beautiful country. And I'm sure it's not news to you that most fast-food choices are bad for your health. These meals are usually brimming with artery-clogging, heart-attack-causing amounts of calories, fat, and sodium.

Now you may say, "But, Dr. Manny, I get the salad when I go down to my favorite fast-food restaurant!" Well, while most fast-food chains have added healthy or light items to their menus over the past couple of years, you need to check out the whole package and ask yourself these questions: Is it fresh? Does the dressing have a ton of sugar and chemicals in it? Am I really getting the nutrition I need? The answers are probably no, yes, and no.

✔ MONEY

The other excuse I often hear for falling into poor eating habits is the one that includes the bottom line: money. Well, my friend, I'd be the first to tell you that eating healthy ain't always cheap. Let's face it, that whole-grain bread isn't in the bargain rack as much as its bleached-out cousin. That goes for many sugar-packed snacks, not to mention cereals. And oh! I have kids! I know that walking along those cereal aisles can be like walking through a junk-food minefield. If you have children, you know the drill: you go to the supermarket, child in tow, and your seven-year-old child who just saw a commercial for Exploding Sugar O's starts saying he simply *has to* have them. To top it all off, they're the featured cheap cereal of the week—so there are millions of these huge boxes displayed all over the store, basically screaming "buy me" to you and your family.

Well, between your very influential offspring and your wallet, it gets dicey. I don't have to tell you that budgets are much tighter than waistlines; trying to justify buying healthier choices, versus what your pocketbook allows, can be real tough.

✔ TIME

In addition to money, the other commodity many of us are short on is time. I know how it is: you've got a big twenty minutes (or less!) for lunch. Sure, you *try* to make your lunch from time to time. But it's not easy—and there's a place on the corner that offers you a superquick and cheap lunch.

✔ STRESS

"Time for *myself*? What's that?" is the usual response I get when I suggest my overachieving patients take some *me* time. Honestly, I get tired just hearing what my wife, Katarina, does every day! And I'll be the first to tell you that with three kids—and a husband who's not around all the time—she's got a hefty load to carry (and though it could be, that's not a direct reference to *my* weight!).

The fact of the matter is that because moms are so busy being supermoms and running around like maniacs, they're not eating as they should. Having one or more kids to care for, getting them off to school in the morning, getting involved in their after-school activities and sports, not to mention their own work, and being part of the sandwich generation (caring for elderly parents as well) all adds up to crazy schedules, unhealthy eating, and in many cases a seeking of foods that immediately satisfy (chips, brownies, candy, cookies, soda, ice cream) but don't promise benefits in return.

✔ LACK OF EXERCISE OR PHYSICAL ACTIVITY

It's a logical equation really. Ask anyone who's not sleeping what they want to do and I guarantee that working out is going to be at the bottom of the list. The thing about exercise, as I tell my patients, is that yes, it needs to be done, but it has to be something that fits your lifestyle: if you can swing getting up at six to go to a yoga class, going on a bike ride (inside or outside), running on a treadmill, or walking outside for half an hour, then that's what you should do. If not, maybe in the middle of the day—even during a lunch break—would work for you (as long as you're not skipping your lunch). Don't tell me you don't have time; you'll need to make the time. This—again—is for your life! This doesn't mean that it will be easy, but it will help and you will see and feel results physically and mentally—almost immediately.

✔ HORMONES

Ask any woman and you'll hear the same thing: appetites grow and fade depending on the time of the month. Most women I know feel incredibly peckish that week before their period; the stereotype of a woman suffering from PMS as a chocolate searching fiend is not too far from what I've seen. And this snacking often leads to the avalanche effect: when you might start with one cookie, which leads to another, and, well, you get the idea!

✔ SNACKING—THE WRONG WAY!

Most of us parents know that we've got to have the snacks on hand, right? Any trip, whether it's a walk to the park or a drive to the supermarket, requires keeping a few treats nearby—for the kids, that is. Here's the problem: we grown-ups like to snack, too!

Well, we're in good company! Just one walk down the snack section of any supermarket will show you that America loves to munch on all kinds of little salty and sweet things; the choice is really overwhelming and not entirely healthy.

✔ LACK OF SLEEP

Sleep deprivation can also affect appetites—not to mention everything else. It's funny, but my wife is *always* the one who wakes up when one of the kids is up (strange how I've been conditioned to sleep through it all!), and I think that's the case with many women; they're intrinsically wired with a wake-up sensibility. The problem with constantly functioning with a sleep deficiency is, of course, that over time this leads not only to exhaustion, but also to a wearing down of wills—which can manifest itself in late-night sweet-food binges. I can't tell you how many times my patients have confessed late-night affairs with their two favorite men: Ben and Jerry. It's true; the less we sleep, the weaker we are in terms of being able to fend off not only increased emotional sensitivity, but crazy cravings for comfort foods. Also, did you know that sleep patterns can be disturbed by many things that you consume—including food additives and caffeine?

So, after considering these eight factors that contribute to this nationwide epidemic, what should you do? What do you need to change to get yourself to a point where you look good, your skin looks healthy and clear, and most important, you *feel* good—less stressed out—and attractive? I'm not talking about surgery here; what I am talking about is taking a more balanced approach—and a philosophy—that will yield you long-lasting and fabulous results. What this diet will do is help you learn the fundamental and effective ways to balance nutrition, exercise, and health. If you stay on the Hot Latin Diet, you will see changes. You'll have more energy, both physically and emotionally, as soon as seven days after you start. After fourteen days, you'll see less weight, and feel even better. If you follow this diet, in just four more weeks you could decrease your body fat by between 5 and 10 percent, lose up to eight to twelve pounds, see a significant change in your skin and the brightness of your eyes. But most important—you'll feel hot!

UNDERSTANDING FOOD AND NUTRITION

Food and nutrition can become daunting and confusing, especially when so many diets are saying so many different things. The good news is, no matter how you spin it, there is an absolute truth as to which foods are good and which are bad. In order to determine that for yourself, you need to understand the fundamentals of six key elements: carbs, sugars, fats, protein, fiber, and dairy.

THE TRUTH ABOUT CARBS

Carbohydrates (meaning "carbon plus water") are the most efficient fuel for your body. They provide steady healthy energy. Along with fat and protein, carbohydrates are an essential nutrient. The two major forms of carbs are: simple sugars (simple carbohydrates), found in sugars such as fructose, glucose, and lactose, as well as in nutritious whole fruits; and starches (complex carbohydrates), found in foods such as starchy vegetables, grains, rice, and breads and cereals.

What makes carbs different from other essential nutrients (fat and protein) is that they are easily converted to energy by the body. Furthermore, the simplest carbohydrate, glucose, is essential fuel for the brain and muscles. When glucose is absorbed from the intestine into the bloodstream, blood-glucose levels increase, and your pancreas begins to secrete insulin to help get that sugar out of the blood and to the brain and muscles. The problem occurs when too much glucose overwhelms the metabolism. In other words, if you regularly eat great amounts of foods with refined starches and sugars—the bad carbs—the pancreas makes too much insulin and the blood sugar drops too far, which, in turn, makes you feel hungry. Furthermore, muscle cells will stop taking in the glucose, and so more of this sugar will be stored as fat, which will result in weight gain.

THE GLYCEMIC INDEX (GI)

This index is a rating system of carbohydrates based on their immediate effect on our blood-glucose (blood-sugar) levels. Carbs that are converted to glucose very fast have a high GI value. These are the carbs that cause a spike and then a drop in our blood sugar, often causing mood swings, or energy bursts and subsequent lags. Carbs that metabolize slowly, releasing glucose gradually into the bloodstream, have a low GI value; these are better for you because they cause a steadier flow of glucose and subsequently energy. (Nutritional experts now believe that high blood-sugar and insulin levels, caused by overeating high-GI carbs in our diet, are one of the key factors responsible for the rise in heart disease, hypertension, diabetes, and insulin resistance.) Not as commonly known, but proven in medical studies, is that a main culprit in contributing to high cholesterol levels is actually sugar and white flours, even more than high-cholesterol foods!

As a general rule, the more natural and unrefined the carbohydrate is, the healthier it is. Also, the lower the glycemic index (GI) value, the better the carb is for your blood-glucose levels. Unrefined whole-grain carbs that have a low or intermediate GI rating are best. For example:

▶ A low glycemic rating is: 55 points or less

▶ An intermediate glycemic rating is: 55–70

▶ A high glycemic rating is: 70 and higher

BEANS	Glycemic Level
garbanzos	**36**
lentils	29
black beans	28
red kidney beans	29
pinto beans	27

FRUIT	Glycemic Level
mango	56
papaya	57
pineapple	66
cherimoya	53
passion fruit	55
guava	57
açaí	22
lime	23
orange	43
watermelon	53
baby bananas	58

VEGETABLES AND CHILES	Glycemic Index
tomato	30
tomatillo	**30**
plantain	60
yellow onion	41
avocado	**12**
jícama	16

VEGETABLES AND CHILES	Glycemic Index
nopale	16
pumpkin	19
artichoke	15
radish	10
spinach	15
red bell pepper	15
jalapeño	**10**
chipotle	**10**

GRAINS AND TUBERS	Glycemic Index
quinoa	67
amaranth	68
brown rice	55
wild rice	53
corn	60
yuca	60
malanga/yautía	53
camote/boniato	50

Note: *Nuts, oils, seafood, poultry, eggs, meat, herbs, and spices all have very low glycemic ratings and do not directly affect blood sugar, and are therefore not listed on the charts above.*

The glycemic index stays the same regardless of portion size, but if you eat a large amount of any food, it will affect blood-sugar levels and cause weight gain. Basically the glycemic index is a measurement for how quickly and how much sugar gets released into the bloodstream after eating certain foods. The trouble with high glycemic foods is that all the sugar in the blood gets stored in fat cells if it is not processed efficiently by the liver, and also these foods are not available for energy since, unless you are extremely physically active and burn the food right away, they are immediately stored as fat rather than giving you a long, sustained energy release.

To be healthy and lean, and to be able to successfully utilize the calories you ingest for your benefit, it is best to eat foods high in fiber, along with some healthy fats and proteins, as this reduces and slows down the amount of sugar that is released into the blood, making it more available, a little at a time, for energy usage rather than fat storage.

All the seven Latin powerfoods and other foods in the Latin powerfood categories have intermediate to low glycemic ratings, so you are on the right track if you start eating according to my Hot Latin Diet.

GOOD CARB FOODS

Complex carbohydrates are the good carbs. Among good carbs are high-fiber, low-sugar fruits, vegetables, legumes, whole oatmeal and all other whole grains, and all types of beans (a Latin staple!). Sweet potatoes, brown rice, grapefruit, fat-free milk (organic and in moderation, please), whole-grain pasta (also in moderation), and apples, like other good carbs, cause a gradual rise in blood-sugar levels, which is optimal for sustained energy, mental clarity and focus, and a balanced mood. Also, eating good carbs will help curb your cravings for bad carbs, which in turn can help you avoid chemical imbalances in the brain that can cause depression.

Note: I always recommend buying organic products, because they're free of potentially harmful ingredients.

BAD CARB FOODS

Excess consumption of refined carbohydrates (refined sugars found in foods and beverages like candy and soda, and refined grains like white rice and white flour, found in many pastas and breads) are one reason behind the dramatic rise of obesity in the United States. Bad carbs—sugar and refined, processed, frozen, canned, and most packaged, deep-fried, and fast foods—contribute to excess calories without nutritional benefits. Bad carbs are refined, high-sugar, white-flour foods that are quickly digested and cause a rapid rise in blood sugar. This sugar spike causes the body to increase the production of insulin, which tells the body to store extra sugar as fat. Other examples of bad carbs include white bread, bagels, potato and corn chips, French fries, and refined sugary cereals, including those that pose as health cereals—read the ingredient list; sugar is there. (A note on cereals: If they're not in the health-food store, they may not be healthy; stick to our whole-food recipes for breakfast alternatives as much as possible.) Also, you should know that good carbs, such as whole oats and wheat, are often transformed into bad carbs through processing. Traditional oatmeal is far better than its quick-cooking cousin or cold oat cereals or shredded wheat.

Note: Please read the ingredients list on packaged foods. If an ingredients list has items that are hard to pronounce and sound like chemicals, you should avoid that product. Also, any ingredient ending in "-ose" is a sugar, such as: maltose, lactose, sucrose, dextrose, fructose, and high-fructose corn syrup; these should also be avoided. No better are all the artificial sweeteners; avoid these as much as possible. Artificial sweeteners include maltitol, sugar alcohols, xylitol, and saccharin, to name a few.

SUGAR CONTENT

All carbohydrates are technically sugar, though there is a big difference between naturally occurring sucrose in plants and the sucrose found in granulated sugar or the high-fructose corn syrup often used to sweeten processed foods. Before your body will use the carbohydrate in table sugar, a baked potato, or a green bean, it must break this carbohydrate down to glucose, the form of sugar that your body can use for energy. If you have too much glucose in your bloodstream, caused by the ingestion of too many carbohydrates, it will inhibit the body's metabolism from breaking it down. Instead, the sugar will be stored as fat.

The average American consumes a huge amount of sugar, between two and three pounds each week. There are many problems linked to too much blood sugar. Diabetes, in which the body becomes increasingly unable to regulate blood-sugar levels, is one of the most serious conditions. Also, elevated blood sugar, even if you don't suffer from diabetes, elevates your risk of heart disease and pancreatic cancer. There are many other health reasons why you shouldn't have too much sugar, ranging from dental issues (cavities, for example) to the promotion of aging.

Refined sugars are the ones you should avoid. Highly refined sugars come in the form of sucrose (table sugar), dextrose (corn sugar), and high-fructose corn syrup and are processed into many foods, such as bread, breakfast cereals, mayonnaise, peanut butter, ketchup, spaghetti sauce, and many prepared meals.

Many advocate natural brown sugar as a healthier choice. This raw sugar—produced from the first crystallization of cane—is free of the additional dyes and chemicals found in refined table sugar. Sugars of any kind provide about 16 calories per teaspoon (4 calories per gram, or 120 per ounce), but these calories, even from the raw brown sugar, are "empty": they have no nutritional value. Try to avoid snacks/foods/cereals/juices in which sugar is listed among the first of the ingredients, any refined sugar (white sugars, dextrose, and high-fructose corn syrup), and instead take your sugars from naturally occurring sources, such as fruits and vegetables. Also avoid sweeter prepared sauces (such as ketchup and some other prepared marinades and sauces), as well as canned fruits in syrups or sugar.

I recommend no more than 12 grams (1 tablespoon) of sugar per day. Also, if a single serving has close to a tablespoon of sugar in it, it should be considered a dessert! Again, learn what the ingredients are in what you are eating, so you can avoid consuming "hidden" sugars. If you stick to the most natural sources of food, as opposed to processed versions, you will be fine.

THE SKINNY ON FATS

Your recommended daily fat intake will depend on many factors, and you will have to determine for yourself what works for you based on your physical activity levels, your age, your current weight, and your metabolism type and body type.

My approach in this book is to encourage you to relate emotionally and mentally to food the way a traditional Latin person would before the advent of fast food and diets, which is to relax about all the numbers and simply eat balanced, natural meals, take time to enjoy each meal, and do not overeat. But it is always a good idea to know the facts. Please see the chart below to find out how much fat you should limit yourself to per day, just to keep yourself mentally in check.

To help you determine your ideal fat intake, I will give you a simple formula to calculate how much fat to consume daily, but remember that this is for the average of all the factors I have listed in the book. Trust your body—if you eat our balanced meals, in time you will learn to listen to what your body needs and adjust accordingly.

Daily Caloric Intake	Recommended Daily Fat Intake in Calories	In Fat Grams
2,500	375–500	42–56
2,000	300–400	33–44
1,800	270–360	30–40

Basically, your fat intake will be approximately ⅟₇ to ⅕ of your daily food and calorie intake. As you can see, there is a large range per daily caloric intake, and this will depend on your unique body composition. Do not be afraid to eat fats—healthy fats like the ones in my charts, that is. Healthy fats can actually speed up your metabolism and support your body to burn more fat.

One more important note: Beyond Track One you do not need to eat less than 1,800 calories a day to lose weight. This will just slow down your metabolism in the long run and most likely cause you to overeat down the line. A standard caloric intake for a woman is 2,000 a day, 2,500 if you are quite physically active, exercising daily. The Hot Latin Diet is a lifestyle, not a crash diet.

GOOD FATS VERSUS BAD FATS

The Hot Latin Diet is about eating healthy and well-rounded meals, and not about excluding fat. But the only type of fat I recommend eating is good: healthy, natural fat from plants, such as vegetable oils and raw nuts, and a small amount of fat from lean meats. Also, keep in mind the health risks involved with eating processed high-fat foods: cancer, diabetes, high cholesterol, and heart disease, among other illnesses. Healthy fats, in moderation, of course, will actually support your brain function, your immune and nervous system, and keep you energized.

On the other hand bad fats, meaning saturated and *trans* fats, have been determined to increase the risk for certain diseases while good fats, meaning monounsaturated and polyunsaturated fats, lower the risk. Again, the key is to substitute good fats for bad fats.

There are medical reasons as to why we need some fat in our diet. If we don't have it, we can't absorb vitamins A, D, E, and K, which are all fat-soluble. Certain types of fat, our essential fatty acids, are crucial for good health. Essential fatty acids (EFAs) are necessary fats that humans cannot synthesize, and can only be obtained through diet. EFAs support the reproductive, immune, cardiovascular, and nervous systems. We need EFAs to manufacture and repair cell membranes, enabling the cells to obtain optimum nutrition and expel harmful waste products. Also, good fats raise your good cholesterol (HDL). One of the jobs of this high-density lipoprotein (HDL) is to take your bad cholesterol, LDL (low-density lipoprotein), to the liver, where it is broken down and excreted. In other words, these good fats remedy some of the damage done by the bad fats.

A primary function of EFAs is the production of prostaglandins, which regulate body functions, such as heart rate, blood pressure, blood clotting, fertility, and conception. They're also very important for our immune systems because they regulate inflammation and encourage the body to fight infection. Pregnant and nursing women's adequate supply of EFAs are also very important for their growing fetus and child.

The problem, however, is that the average U.S. diet contains too much total fat, especially saturated and trans fat, which is associated with increased rates of heart disease and stroke. All fat contains 9 calories per gram, more than twice as many calories as carbohydrates (and protein).

Good Fats: Found in salmon, mackerel, sardines, anchovies, albacore tuna, and other seafoods, canola oil (cold-pressed and unrefined), soybean oil, flaxseed oil, olive oil (extra-virgin or virgin), olives, avocados, walnuts, pumpkin seeds, Brazil nuts, almonds, peanuts, sesame oil, pecans, pistachio nuts, cashews, hazelnuts, and macadamia nuts, good fats are the naturally occurring, traditional fats that haven't been damaged by high heat, refining, processing, or other man-made tampering, such as partial hydrogenation. Animal fats have a bad reputation, but many professionals believe it is not animal fat, but the combination of animal foods, fats and low-fiber vegetables that is the problem.

Bad Fats: The worst type of fat is the man-made trans fats, like those found in hydrogenated or partially hydrogenated oils (these oils have been processed with high heat, which removes all the healthy nutrients), refined vegetable oils like margarine, nondairy creamers, and shortening. These are also found in cakes, icings, cookies, donuts, and potato chips. Trans fats negatively impact not only your waistline, but also your nervous system and blood vessels. Bad fats also include saturated fats, like bacon and bacon grease, butter (stick, whipped, and reduced fat), cream, half-and-half, cream cheese, ice cream, lard, salt pork, and palm and palm kernel oil. Eaten in its natural state, coconut, though a saturated fat, is not a bad fat since it comes from plant origin. In fact, it offers many medicinal and immune-boosting properties. Coconut water is nature's best sports drink, because the water resembles the plasma component of our blood in mineral content. In fact, I recommend drinking good-quality water—or coconut water—over any juice or sports drink. In general, you should limit your saturated-fat intake to less than 7 percent of your daily calories. Anything with trans fat should be avoided entirely.

Note: Because of factory farming methods, antibiotics, and steroid use, fats from non–organically raised, non-free-range animals should be avoided.

According to the World Health Organization (WHO) we should restrict our dietary fat intake to 30 percent of our calories. Heart associations suggest 20–30 percent, while some experts believe that we may actually need as little as 10 percent of our calories in the form of fat. However, again, fat quantity is not the only issue: the type of fat is also important. Certain types of fats (for example omega-3 fats) from whole foods like nuts, seeds, and oily fish are now viewed as essential to a healthy diet.

For optimum health and weight loss, you need to reduce your overall fat consumption to a sensible level, and restrict your consumption of saturated fat, and definitely eliminate all trans fats from your diet. Food labels list trans fat content on them; steer clear when you see hydrogenated oil or partially hydrogenated oil listed as ingredients.

Note: Combining healthy carbs with a little bit of fat and protein is a balanced way to nourish your body and increase your metabolism. The addition of protein and healthy fat to a meal helps to reduce the glycemic impact on your body, and makes for a more sustained energy supply.

PROTEIN

Adequate protein intake is crucial for good health. It plays a fundamental role in practically all biological processes in the body. All enzymes are proteins and are vital for the body's metabolism. Proteins facilitate muscle contraction, immune protection, and the transmission of nerve impulses. Proteins in skin and bone provide structural support. Protein is an important part of every diet and is found in many different foods. Some of the protein you eat contains all the amino acids needed to build new proteins. This kind is called complete protein. (Animal sources of protein are usually complete.) Other protein sources may be missing one or more amino acids that the body can't make from scratch or create by modifying another amino acid. Called incomplete proteins, these usually come from fruits, vegetables, grains, and nuts.

I suggest varying your protein sources rather than sticking to, let's say, chicken all the time. One thing about Latinos is that they love flavor and variety! The approximate recommended daily allowance of protein is not as high as you may think. Most women require only 47 grams of protein daily, and most men require 54 grams daily. Most people eat way more protein than their bodies actually need to stay healthy. I suggest you spread out your protein intake throughout the day, combined with healthy carbohydrates and fats, like a balanced meal or snack. This is the traditional Latin way, just like in the delicious recipes created by our fabulous chefs.

Lean proteins are the best kind. These can be found in fish, skinless chicken and turkey, pork tenderloin, and certain cuts of beef, like the top round. Low-fat dairy products like milk, yogurt, ricotta and other cheeses supply both protein and calcium. As far as vegetarians or vegans are concerned, if you don't eat meat, fish, poultry, eggs, or dairy products, you need to eat a variety of protein-containing foods each day—for example, tofu, chickpeas, lentils, soy milk, peanuts, and bread. Eggs, cows' milk, and hard cheese—for dairy-eating vegetarians—have a good amount of protein per individual serving (between 6 and 9 grams).

Some Other Good Sources of Protein

Wild (Not Farmed) Fish: offers heart-healthy omega-3 fatty acids and, in general, less fat than meat.

Organic (Free-Range) Poultry: provides high protein, and is leaner than meat. You can get rid of most of the saturated fat by removing the skin.

Beans: contain more protein than any other vegetable. (And they're packed with fiber that helps you feel full for hours.)

Nuts: one ounce of almonds gives you 6 grams of protein, nearly as much protein as one ounce of broiled rib eye steak.

Whole grains: a slice of whole-wheat bread gives you 3 grams of protein, plus valuable fiber.

Note: To create a complete protein from vegetarian sources, you will need to mix grains with protein—for example, whole-grain sprouted bread with almond butter.

FIBER

Dietary fiber slows the rise in blood sugar, gives you energy, and keeps you satisfied longer by slowing gastric emptying, which leads to an overall decrease in calorie intake. It's associated with decreased cardiovascular risk and a slower progression of cardiovascular disease in high-risk individuals, especially when eaten regularly as part of a diet low in saturated fat, trans fat, and cholesterol. Fiber also aids in removing waste from your intestines and making your bowel movements regular. Thanks to fiber, impurities are pulled out of your digestive system, helping you to lose weight and detoxify at the same time. A food is high in fiber if it has at least 5 grams per serving. The Institute of Medicine recommends consuming 14 grams of fiber for every 1,000 calories you need, so that's about 28 grams a day.

Some Foods High in Fiber

Grain Products

whole-grain breads	whole grains, such as:
some bran cereals	quinoa
oatmeal	barley
whole-wheat pastas	corn
	brown rice

Fruits

dried fruits, such as:	berries, such as:
apricots	blackberries
dates	blueberries
prunes	raspberries
raisins (be sure to get the ones without the preservative sulfur dioxide)	strawberries

(continued)

Some Foods High in Fiber (continued)

Fruits (continued)

avocados	apples (with skin)
oranges	kiwis

Vegetables

broccoli	green peas
spinach	other dark green leafy vegetables
Swiss chard	

Beans

dried peas

beans, such as:

garbanzos (chickpeas)	black-eyed beans
kidney beans	lentils
lima beans	

Nuts and Seeds

almonds	soy nuts
whole flaxseed	

Note: These foods contain more than 5 grams per serving. Organic products are always preferable.

Be sure to read labels carefully: Many commercial oat bran and wheat bran products (muffins, chips, waffles) contain very little bran. Also, it's important to note that fiber by itself, without the necessary water intake, doesn't do much for your diet. In fact, when not taken with enough water, fiber will cause constipation by soaking up water already in your body. In order to make sure you reap the most benefits from your fiber, make sure to drink about two liters of water (minimum) a day. The old minimum of eight glasses of water a day translates into about two liters.

DAIRY

It is important for women to have calcium because of the role it plays in bone development. Adequate amounts of this mineral will help you reach optimum amounts of bone density, which will help protect you from osteoporosis later in life, and prevent the breakdown of bone. Furthermore, it's been found that calcium may also prevent PMS. The amount of calcium that a woman should get per day ranges from 1,000 to 1,500 milligrams, depending on age group and hormonal state.

Dairy products are a good source of calcium, but they're also full of fat (and inappropriate for women who are lactose intolerant, vegan, or allergic—or have religious or other self-imposed dietary restrictions). If you do eat/drink dairy, make sure to choose organic and lower-fat options. In any case, it's important to vary the sources of calcium intake. Contrary to popular belief, dairy is not the ideal source of calcium, be-cause though dairy itself may have high levels of the mineral, this cal-cium doesn't absorb into human bodies so well. This is clearly evidenced by the epidemic of osteoporosis we have in this country, despite huge amounts of dairy consumption. In fact, there are plenty of cultures worldwide that don't consume dairy but have strong teeth and bones.

For calcium to be optimally absorbed in your body, you must also take a calcium supplement along with vitamin C, a mineral complex supplement, and essential fatty acids. Some excellent sources of cal-cium (a good source of calcium contributes approximately 100 mil-ligrams of calcium in a standard serving) beyond dairy foods include:

- leafy green vegetables like broccoli, beet greens, mustard greens, kale, and spinach

- fruit like dried figs and oranges

- beans and peas

- tofu, peanuts, black beans, baked beans

- fish like salmon and sardines

- nuts and seeds like sesame seeds and almonds

Calcium is also found in blackstrap molasses, corn tortillas, and some brown sugar.

MYTH BUSTERS

Because there is so much conflicting health information in the media, you may have your own stigmas associated with certain foods. Below are some myth busters to address some common misconceptions about nutrition.

Myth: Fruit Juices Are High in Carbs and Low in Fiber.

Juices do, in fact, have redeeming qualities for your health, and there are times when juice is uniquely beneficial. After a workout, for example, it helps replace fluids and blood sugar and provides nutrients. Juice also comes in handy when eating is simply not convenient—when you're driving, say, or traveling, but still want something with nutritional value. Be sure to drink 100 percent juice, with no added sweeteners, or no sugar added. But be careful; the calories quickly add up!

Myth: Ketosis Is Good for You.

This is definitely misleading. Ketosis is a sign that the blood is becoming too acidic. To combat this, the body takes calcium from the bones, which raises the risk of osteoporosis. In fact, the Nurses' Health Study showed that women on higher-protein diets had a higher risk of bone fractures. Ketosis can also damage the kidneys, cause bad breath, and trigger irregular heart rhythms that can cause sudden death.

Myth: Eggs Are Bad for You.

A study published in 1999 that followed thirty-eight thousand men and eighty thousand women found that an egg a day had no impact on the risk of heart disease or stroke in healthy men and women. Eggs eaten in moderation, about three or four a week, are fine for most people. Health professionals advise people who already have high blood cholesterol to carefully watch their saturated fat intake and lose weight if they are overweight.

Myth: Taking Vitamins Replaces the Need for Healthy Foods.

So-called whole foods like veggies and whole grains contain fiber and a host of other important nutrients that can't be adequately delivered through pills. In fact, scientists are still finding new "trace elements" in whole foods that may someday be labeled essential to health—but aren't found in any pill. Many experts will tell you that taking vitamins doesn't compensate for a healthy diet.

FOODS THAT HELP YOUR BODY FIGHT!

Now let's focus on doctor-recommended foods that help potentially safeguard you from harmful diseases and pump up your immune system.

Foods That Fight Arthritis: salmon, bananas, sweet peppers, shrimp, soy products, sweet potatoes, cheese, lentils, green tea

Foods That Can Stop a Heart Attack: foods high in potassium, like fat-free and 1% milk, low-fat yogurt, vegetable juice cocktail, baby limas, kidney beans, and lentils

Foods That Fight or Prevent Heart Disease: oats, soy, legumes, garlic, apples, oranges, grapefruits and most fruits, walnuts, green leafy vegetables, carrots, sweet potatoes, and cantaloupes

Foods That Fight Cancer: folate-rich foods, vitamin D, tea, cruciferous vegetables, curcumin, and ginger

Foods That Fight Aging: Experts suspect the antioxidant compounds found in produce, legumes, and whole grains are largely responsible for holding back the march of time.

UNDERSTANDING YOUR BODY

We all know when we should lose weight, right? We sometimes determine we need to lose weight based on various measurements, one of which is your BMI, your body mass index—a measurement of your body fat based on your height and weight. The BMI is one type of indication that, under certain circumstances, can tell you if you are underweight, normal, overweight, or obese. For adults who are twenty years of age or older, they can calculate their BMI with this formula: BMI $=$ (Weight in pounds / [Height in inches] $\times$ [Height in inches]) $\times$ 703, or you can use one of the many online calculators, such as the one at www. nhlbisupport .com/bmi/. Having a BMI of 25 or higher indicates being overweight; and being below the healthy range (18.5 to 24.9) can indicate a potential health problem.

It's important to note that although BMI is accurate most of the time, it doesn't work for all of us, doesn't take all body types into account, and may overestimate or underestimate body fat. For example, BMI doesn't distinguish between body fat and muscle mass, which weighs more than fat. So many professional athletes—like football players—would be mislabeled as obese according to this scale because of their high BMI, when they actually have a low percentage of body fat.

BMI CHART

BMI	19	20	21	22	23	24	25	26	27	28	29	30	35	40
Height						Weight (lbs.)								
4'10"	91	96	100	105	110	115	119	124	129	134	138	143	167	191
4'11"	94	99	104	109	114	119	124	128	133	138	143	148	173	198
5'0"	97	102	107	112	118	123	128	133	138	143	148	153	179	204
5'1"	100	106	111	116	122	127	132	137	143	148	153	158	185	211
5'2"	104	109	115	120	126	131	136	142	147	153	158	164	191	218
5'3"	107	113	118	124	130	135	141	146	152	158	163	169	197	225
5'4"	110	116	122	128	134	140	145	151	157	163	169	174	204	232
5'5"	114	120	126	132	138	144	150	156	162	168	174	180	210	240
5'6"	118	124	130	136	142	148	155	161	167	173	179	186	216	247
5'7"	121	127	134	140	146	153	159	166	172	178	185	191	223	255
5'8"	125	131	138	144	151	158	164	171	177	184	190	197	230	262
5'9"	128	135	142	149	155	162	169	176	182	189	196	203	236	270
5'10"	132	139	146	153	160	167	174	181	188	195	202	207	243	278
5'11"	136	143	150	157	165	172	179	186	193	200	208	215	250	286
6'0"	140	147	154	162	169	177	184	191	199	206	213	221	258	294
6'1"	144	151	159	166	174	182	189	197	204	212	219	227	265	302
6'2"	148	155	163	171	179	186	194	202	210	218	225	233	272	311
6'3"	152	160	168	176	184	192	200	208	216	224	232	240	279	319
6'4"	156	164	172	180	189	197	205	213	221	230	238	246	287	328

BMI Classification

18.5 or less	Underweight
18.5 to 24.99	Normal Weight
25 to 29.99	Overweight
30 to 34.99	Obesity (Class 1)
35 to 39.99	Obesity (Class 2)
40 or greater	Morbid Obesity

In thinking about weight, I wanted to include another point of reference. This next chart, which applies solely to women (the weight chart for men is different), is just to give you some ballpark figures for you to check out in relation to your own height and weight, according to your frame.

WEIGHT IN POUNDS, BASED ON AGES 25–59, WITH THE LOWEST MORTALITY RATE			
Height	**Small Frame**	**Medium Frame**	**Large Frame**
4'10"	102–111	109–121	118–131
4'11"	103–113	111–123	120–134
5'0"	104–115	113–126	122–137
5'1"	106–118	115–129	125–140
5'2"	108–121	118–132	128–143
5'3"	111–124	121–135	131–147
5'4"	114–127	124–138	134–151
5'5"	117–130	127–141	137–155
5'6"	120–133	130–144	140–159
5'7"	123–136	133–147	143–163
5'8"	126–139	136–150	146–167
5'9"	129–142	139–153	149–170
5'10"	132–145	142–156	152–173
5'11"	135–148	145–159	155–176
6'0"	138–151	148–162	158–179

Source: www.healthchecksystems.com/heightweightchart.htm

Note: These calculations include indoor clothing weighing three pounds and shoes with one-inch heels.

CALORIES

Ideally you are getting aerobic exercise a minimum of three times a week for at least thirty minutes each session (this would put you in the moderately active category; active would be between five and seven times a week). There is a simple formula to determine your daily caloric needs:

For women who are sedentary: weight $\times$ 14 = estimated calories/day.

For women who are moderately active: weight $\times$ 17 = estimated calories/day.

For women who are active: weight $\times$ 20 = estimated calories/day.

MUSCLE VERSUS FAT

Facts on fat:

▶ Fat is only reduced when you burn more calories than you consume in a day. If you don't burn more calories than you consume, you will gain weight.

▶ Fat does not turn into muscle and muscle cannot become fat. (They have two totally different structures and functions, and react in different ways.)

▶ Fat will not increase if you stop training, and start eating less.

▶ Fat may increase if you begin training and also increase the amount you're eating.

▶ You can't choose where to lose or gain weight on your body.

Because muscles use more calories than fat—even while you're resting—it's good to build stronger muscles, which can happen through exercise, with or without weights. The reason this happens is because exercise contributes to having a faster and more efficient metabolism; your body will burn energy more efficiently if it's in good shape.

ANOTHER MEASUREMENT: WHR

The waist–hip ratio (or waist-to-hip ratio) is the ratio of the circumference of the waist to that of the hips. It measures the proportion by which fat is distributed around the torso.

Carrying weight around the waist (we also call that the apple-type body) means you have a much higher risk of cardiovascular disease than those who carry weight around the hips (a pear-type body). For cardiovascular diseases, it is less about how overweight you are and more about how your fat is distributed. Particularly harmful are the fat deposits in the waist area and on the internal organs. In fact, internal belly fat has a significant effect on metabolism, because it has a different composition than bottom, hip, or thigh fat; it produces large amounts of fatty acids that are converted into other fats in the liver. Weight gain in internal belly fat thus also increases the risk of secondary diseases.

You can calculate your WHR yourself. Using nonstretchable tape, measure your waist at its narrowest point width-wise (usually just above the belly button) by tightening it without depressing the skin. Then measure your hips around the widest part of the hip bones. Divide the waist measurement by the hip measurement. A WHR of 0.7 for the average woman is ideal because it means that your waist is smaller than your hips and you're not carrying the unhealthiest (riskiest) type of weight around your midsection (that's the area that can lead to heart disease and other diseases). A measurement above 0.7 for WHR may mean a larger midsection, and anything below 0.7 means a narrower waist compared to hips; this is what you should aim for. Women around the 0.7 WHR have optimal levels of estrogen and are less susceptible to such major diseases as diabetes, cardiovascular disorders, and ovarian cancers.

Your Goals

Now that you've learned about weight gain, food and nutrition, and your body, and have some numbers and ranges, what should you shoot for? You know that this is a lifestyle change that requires many different ways of looking at food, as well as exercise. Below are long-term goals to work toward while on the Hot Latin Diet. These are designed to help you monitor your progress effectively and maintain the results well beyond the last track of the plan. As for short-term goals, there are two key components we will measure against at the end of each track: weight and body fat.

Here Are Key Target Goals to Follow While You Are on the Hot Latin Diet:

1. Reach for a BMI within a range of 18.5 to 24.9.

2. Work toward a WHR of 0.7.

3. Monitor your caloric intake during the first two tracks. You should limit your calories to 1,500 to 1,800 a day for Track One, and then move gradually to 1,800 to 2,000 calories a day for Track Two.

4. Limit total fat consumption to 30 percent of your total calories.

5. Reserve 20 percent of your total calories for lean protein.

6. During the day, select most of your carbs from the low-to-intermediate glycemic levels (55 to 70 points). During the

night, try to limit your carb consumption to foods only in the low glycemic level (55 points or less).

(7) You should consume at least 28 grams of fiber per day.

(8) Eat three small meals and two snacks per day. (Make sure to eat a satisfying breakfast and try to eat dinner before eight p.m.)

(9) Drink a minimum of eight glasses of water per day, which translates into about two liters.

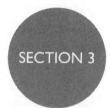

SECTION 3

THE FAST-TRACK PLAN

☑ *Track One: The First Two Weeks*

☑ *Track Two: The Next Four Weeks*

☑ *Track Three: Week Seven and Beyond*

Before you turn the page to get started on your fast- track plan to a slimmer you, I want you to think about a couple of things. First, I want you to maintain this positive feeling of anticipation for as long as you can. Remember, you're doing something great for yourself, and even though this diet will become an everyday thing, I always want you to be able to reach back and feel that on-the-verge-of-something-new feeling—this will help keep you motivated and on track throughout the duration of the diet. Remember, this is something you're doing for yourself, and the success you achieve will depend on your level of commitment and dedication to this new and healthy way of life.

WHAT'S ABOUT TO HAPPEN

Because of the components in the seven Latin powerfoods and other Latin flavors in the powerfood categories, your body will become antioxidized, strong, and nourished. This diet is designed to help you feel full while staying healthy, and you'll quickly start to notice how you no longer feel heavy and sluggish after meals—instead you'll find that you have more energy than before! As you start to incorporate the seven Latin powerfoods into your diet over the next several weeks, your metabolism will begin to function more efficiently, burning more calories and thus getting rid of excess fat.

RECIPE-READING TIPS
....

I don't want to hear the words "I can't cook!" because, my friend, anyone can cook. Well, if you can read, you can cook! Here are a few tips for those of you who are feeling a bit insecure in the kitchen domain. Remember, please, cooking is a skill—which means that just like playing the piano or your favorite game, you *can* get better at it. But, just as my piano teacher always told me, there's only one way to get better: practice, practice, practice! In the meantime, here are some tips to get you started.

(1) Read the recipe! Read it—*all of it*—carefully. Make sure you have all the ingredients in the ingredients list (look at my pantry list, as well as the recipes, for the first two weeks!).

(2) Take out the tools you'll need. For example, do you need a can opener? Blender? Spatula? Sauté pan? Line 'em all up—and keep 'em ready for use.

(3) Check the procedure to see if you need to preheat your oven. Typically an oven should be heated for about fifteen minutes (until it reaches the target temperature).

(4) Look over the preparation of the different ingredients. Does the garlic need to be minced? The tomatoes chopped? Read the chef's suggestions, and follow them! Then set up your prepared ingredients in little bowls or measuring cups (come on—I know you've seen this on TV!) so that you can add them as needed.

(5) Now that you have all your ingredients prepared, read the recipe one more time. Do this for two reasons: first, to make sure you haven't forgotten anything, and second, so that you're that much more familiar with how and when you'll incorporate everything into your dish.

(6) Have fun with it all—and get help as needed! Everyone could use a prep cook in the kitchen, but, alas, it's not a luxury we usually have, so, my friend, it's up to you! Put on some music, and start chopping!

And finally, just one point to finish with. Even if you're new to this whole cooking thing, you're not new to following instructions! Think about what you're doing—have fun with it, and remember, some of the best chefs will tell you that their most innovative recipes have come from making errors. So *por favor*, please, don't be afraid to make a mistake; it's all part of this exciting learning process!

Track One: The First Two Weeks

Feeling better is just one of the primary considerations in choosing the recipes you'll find in the following pages. As I mentioned before, the reason you'll feel better is because of the ingestion of the Latin power-foods, which will help your body function at an optimal level by flushing out the toxins from your cells and allowing them to work efficiently. The recipes listed for the first two weeks were chosen because of the inclusion of more raw salads as well as cooked vegetables, and for their simplicity in terms of ingredients and preparation. Speeding up your body's metabolic function and increasing your weight loss was another key consideration. Track One offers several seafood and fish dishes; this kind of animal protein is easier to digest. Also, for our vegetarian friends, these dishes are certainly adaptable and can be prepared with alternate sources of protein, such as beans or tofu—which will make the dishes even lighter on the body.

What's not a main factor in Track One meals is fat content. In fact, I do not believe in fat-free as indicating healthier eating or causing more weight loss. Actually, the body needs healthy fats in order to burn fat! That's why those fat-free diets do not work—they actually lead to higher blood-sugar levels and cravings for starches, causing the weight to come back on as soon as the diet is over.

Eat five times a day: breakfast, snack, lunch, snack, dinner. The goal for these first two weeks is to consume an average of 1,500 to 1,800 calories a day. Although this may not seem like much, you will be surprised to find that the meals are so satisfying that you won't be starving throughout the day. In fact, I deeply encourage you to *not* starve yourself during this diet, and to eat between meals. That's why among the suggested recipes you'll find a series of healthy snacks that you can consume any time you feel your energy is getting lower—as midmorning or mid-afternoon pick-me-ups. During these first two weeks, you should expect to lose anywhere from four to six pounds. Sound too good to be true? Well, you better believe it! Although a great part of this weight loss will be due to the flushing out of toxins and excess water, the key here is that you are reeducating your body to work more efficiently by giving it the right foods at the right time. You will notice that in Track One I have placed a great emphasis on seafood—with the delicious Tuna Niçoise Salad, which I recommend that you have for lunch, or the Shrimp with Mango-Ginger Sauce, which makes for a great dinner that can be enjoyed by the entire family. The beauty of seafood is that not only is it rich in flavor, but it is also a great source of protein without the high amounts of saturated fat that can be present in other meat products.

The recipes included here are meant to serve as guidelines to what you should be eating during these two first weeks. While they are tasty options to stay on track, remember that you can always mix them up and develop your own, using, of course, the seven Latin powerfoods. Here are a few things you need to keep in mind when crafting your own meals.

BREAKFAST

Not only is this the most important meal of the day, it's also the one where you can get the most creative. In the morning, you need as much energy as you can get, and eating a tasty, satisfying meal will help you fight unnecessary cravings before lunch. So this is the time to load up on your proteins and carbs without feeling guilty; by eating them early in the morning you'll make sure you burn them as you go about your hectic day. Good examples are eggs, toast (always whole grain; stay away from that white bread), and even rice and beans, as you'll see in the Gallo Pinto recipe. It is also a good idea to have a piece of fruit, which will give you the fiber and vitamins you need to be at your peak.

LUNCH

As I mentioned above, the focus for Track One is seafood. Have it as often as you can, and you'll see what a great variety there really is! Just a drizzle of olive oil or a few drops of lemon juice can be enough to spruce up any kind of seafood, and the health benefits are remarkable. Not only does eating fish lower your risk of heart disease, but the omega-3 fatty acids will contribute to making your skin look great!

DINNER

A good alternative to seafood in Track One is poultry, a great source of vitamins and low-fat protein. Because your metabolism slows down in the evening, avoid eating carbs (leave the rice and potatoes for lunchtime!) and instead accompany your meals with a hefty green salad seasoned with a little olive oil, salt, pepper, and lemon to taste.

These delicious and nutritious recipes are well balanced and include a variety of powerfoods from all the food groups we recommend eating. Healthy fats, such as those from lean meats, vegetable oils, and nuts (not from fried and processed foods!) actually are your best source of fuel for steady energy and increased mental focus and clarity throughout your day.

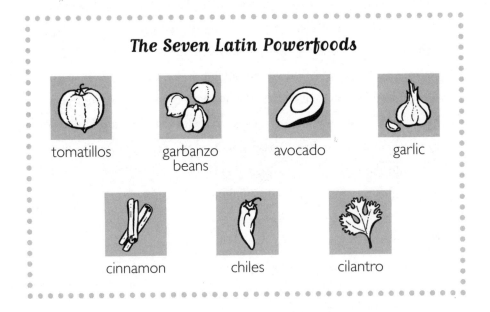

The Seven Latin Powerfoods

tomatillos · garbanzo beans · avocado · garlic

cinnamon · chiles · cilantro

Gallo Pinto, Costa Rican—Style Rice and Beans—Breakfast

CHEF: ARLEN GARGAGLIANO   SERVES 4

● ●

LATIN POWER-FOODS

Any visitor to Costa Rica will learn about breakfast Tico-style—which always includes Gallo Pinto. This can be enjoyed throughout the day, of course, but the Costa Ricans consider it a breakfast first and foremost! Gallo Pinto is made differently from home to home; this comes from Arlen's stay at her friend's casa in San José. As Vivian Vargas taught her, the best rice to use for this dish is leftover white rice, but here we recommend the nutritionally richer choice of brown rice. This dish has two of my Latin powerfoods: garlic and cilantro. It also has bell peppers, onion, black beans, and brown rice.

- 2 tablespoons olive oil

- 2 cloves of garlic, minced

- $^1/_2$ teaspoon fresh ginger, minced (or according to taste)

- ½ red onion, chopped

- 1 red bell pepper, chopped

- 1½ cups of cooked and drained black beans (if you make the beans, save the bean stock)

- 1½ cups of cooked brown rice, at room temperature or warm

- 1 tablespoon Salsa Lizano (available in Latin markets or online) or Worcestershire sauce

- kosher salt and freshly ground black pepper

- 2 tablespoons fresh chopped cilantro leaves

Heat the olive oil in a medium saucepan over medium-high heat (until the oil is hot, but not smoking). Add the garlic, ginger, and onion and cook, stirring frequently. (Lower the heat if the onion starts to brown.) After the onion starts to wilt, about 2 minutes, add the red pepper and sauté until softened, about another 3 minutes. Add the beans, and cook just until the beans warm, about 2 more minutes. Turn off the heat and set aside. Pour the rice into a large bowl. Stir in the bean mixture and mix well. Add the Salsa Lizano (or Worcestershire) and mix well. Add salt and pepper to taste. Stir in the cilantro, and serve—with or without scrambled eggs and a side dish of fresh fruit (preferably tropical!).

Nutritional information per 1-person serving:

	Serving	Calories	Total Fat	Carbs.	Fiber	Sugars	Protein	Antioxidant Rating
Gallo Pinto	1 cup	228	8g	32.5g	7.8g	1g	7.5g	2
Scrambled eggs	3	200	14g	1g	0	0	16g	0
Tropical fruit	1 cup	80	0	19g	1g	10g	1g	2

Spicy Frittata, Tomato Salad—Breakfast

CHEF: MICHELLE BERNSTEIN   SERVES 4

● ●

It would be such a shame to replace such luscious possibilities for breakfasts—like this one—with cereals from a box! This combination of ingredients is sure to get you, and your metabolism, off to a great start. Chef Michelle Bernstein suggests that this breakfast be served with a side dish of warmed black beans topped with a dollop of sour cream. This dish contains the Latin powerfoods chiles (habanero or Scotch bonnet peppers) and cilantro, as well as eggs, onions, kale (or spinach), and tomatoes.

4 large whole eggs

4 egg whites

2 tablespoons fresh parsley, chopped

kosher salt and black pepper to taste

1 tablespoon olive oil

1 cup Spanish onions, peeled, finely chopped

1 cup kale or spinach, sliced thin

¼ piece of habanero or Scotch bonnet pepper, finely diced

1 cup tomatoes, chopped

¼ cup red onion, chopped

½ cup cilantro, chopped

juice of 1 lime

Whisk the whole eggs, egg whites, parsley, salt, and pepper. Set aside.

In a heavy nonstick broiler-proof pan, heat the oil over medium heat. Add the Spanish onion and cook until soft, about 8 minutes. Add the kale and cook for 4 minutes. Stir in the egg mixture and pepper and mix well. Cover with foil and reduce the heat to low and cook until the eggs are almost set, about 6 to 7 minutes.

Meanwhile, prepare the tomato topping: In a food processor, combine the tomato, red onion, cilantro, lime juice, and salt and pepper. Pulse about 5 times, until the mixture resembles a salsa.

Preheat the broiler. Place the frittata under the broiler and cook until the top is set and starts to brown, about 2 to 3 minutes. Place a large serving plate over the pan, and carefully invert to turn out the frittata to serve. Top with the tomato mixture and serve immediately.

Nutritional information per 1-person serving:

	Serving	Calories	Total Fat	Carbs.	Fiber	Sugars	Protein	Antioxidant Rating
Frittata with Tomato Salad	1 cup	147	9.3g	6g	2g	3g	14.6	2
Side of ½ cup black beans with a dollop of sour cream		156	3.5g	22.5	5g	0	9.4g	1

Grilled Tuna Niçoise—Lunch

CHEF: MICHELLE BERNSTEIN   SERVES 4

● ●

LATIN POWER-FOODS

Chef Bernstein insists on using the best-quality tuna for this salad. Her interpretation of the classic French salad has New World touches, making it healthy, colorful, and very tasty. This recipe includes one of my Latin powerfoods, garlic, and tomatoes and eggs.

¼ cup red wine vinegar

2 tablespoons Dijon mustard

1 tablespoon shallots, minced

1 teaspoon garlic, minced

1¼ cup olive oil

salt and pepper

1 Yukon Gold potato, peeled and diced small (¼-inch pieces)

2 cups French beans, trimmed

four 6-ounce sushi-grade tuna fillets

½ cup red onion, peeled, sliced into thin strips (place in ice water, drain, and repeat 3 times)

1 cup red teardrop or grape-size tomatoes

2 cups frisée lettuce

1 cup fennel bulb, sliced very thin (using a Japanese mandolin if available)

4 quail eggs, boiled, peeled, halved

¼ cup small Niçoise olives, pitted

*T*o prepare the vinaigrette, combine the vinegar, mustard, shallots, and garlic in a blender. Purée and slowly drizzle ¼ cup of the olive oil. Season with salt and pepper. Refrigerate until ready to serve.

To cook the potatoes, place a small pot of water on high heat, season with salt. Add the potatoes and cook for 2 to 3 minutes or until cooked through. Remove the potatoes with a slotted spoon (don't pour the water out), and place the potatoes in ice water.

Place the French beans in the same water you cooked the potatoes in (if you've turned the pot of water off, make sure it's on and simmering before you add the beans). Cook until just done but still crisp (be sure not to overcook), between 2 and 3 minutes. Remove from the boiling water and immediately place into ice water to stop the cooking process.

Heat a grill to medium-high heat. Rub the remaining oil, with salt and pepper according to your liking, into the tuna. Set aside until you've prepped the salad. In a large mixing bowl, combine the cooked French beans, potatoes, rinsed and drained onion, tomatoes, frisée lettuce, and fennel. Add the vinaigrette (1 tablespoon at a time) until desired. Mix until well blended. Place a quarter of the salad on each dish. Garnish each plate with the eggs and olives. Place the tuna on the grill and cook just 45 seconds per side. Remove the fillets from the grill, and slice them into five slices each. Place the tuna slices on the prepared salads, and serve immediately.

Nutritional information per 1-person serving:

	Serving	Calories	Total Fat	Carbs.	Fiber	Sugars	Protein	Antioxidant Rating
Whole dish including quail eggs and olives		475	19g	24g	6g	4.9g	55.3g	3
Grilled Tuna	6 ounces	220	6g	0	0	0	50.5g	1
1 cup French salad with ¼ cup vinaigrette		200	9g	23.5g	5.1g	4.9g	3.6g	3

Ceviche—Lunch

CHEF: XIOMARA ARDOLINA   SERVES 4

● ●

LATIN POWER-FOODS

This refreshing lunchtime treat is chef Xiomara Ardolina's interpretation of a classic Peruvian-born dish, which can be found in many variations throughout the Americas. She likes to serve her ceviche in martini glasses, topped with fresh chunks of avocado.

This recipe contains several Latin powerfoods: chiles, cilantro, and avocado. It also has shrimp, limes, and tomatoes.

2 jalapeño chiles

1 pound rock shrimp (or your favorite medium-size shrimp), peeled, deveined, and cut into ¼-inch dice

¾ pound sea scallops (preferably diver)

¾ cup fresh-squeezed lime juice

½ cup fresh-squeezed orange juice

1 cup fresh-squeezed lemon juice

sugar to taste

1 large tomato, roasted, peeled, seeded, and chopped

½ cup red onion, chopped

¼ cup fresh or canned tomato juice

salt and pepper to taste

1 small bunch fresh cilantro, finely chopped

½ Hass avocado, peeled and seeded, quartered, for garnish

Roast jalapeños over a flame or in a pan until the skin blackens and blisters; place in a bag or sealed container. When peppers have cooled, remove the skin with a paper towel; do not rinse. Seed and chop them.

Combine the shrimp and scallops with the three citrus juices and marinate overnight. Taste for sweetness; add sugar as needed. Add the jalapeño, tomato, red onion, and tomato juice. Season with salt and pepper. Add the cilantro, and garnish with avocado just before serving.

	Serving	Calories	Total Fat	Carbs.	Fiber	Sugars	Protein	Antioxidant Rating
1 cup Ceviche with ⅛ avocado		221	5.8g	12.4g	1.9g	5g	29.6g	3

*S*tar Anise and Ginger-Spiced Chicken with Roast Calabaza and Corn—Dinner

CHEF: MICHELLE BERNSTEIN   SERVES 4

● ●

LATIN POWER-FOODS

As chef Michelle Bernstein shows us here, there are so many wonderful ways to combine spices—and you should enjoy exploring! The flavors of this dish are both enchanting and healthful. This recipe has two Latin powerfoods: cilantro and garlic. It also has calabaza (pumpkin), corn, and chicken.

ROAST CALABAZA AND CORN

2 tablespoons olive oil

2 tablespoons dark brown sugar

pinch cinnamon

1 teaspoon vanilla extract

1 pound calabaza, peeled, seeded, and cut into 2-inch cubes

2 cups corn kernels

¼ cup fresh cilantro leaves, finely chopped

¼ cup fresh Italian parsley leaves, finely chopped

coarse salt and black pepper to taste

CHICKEN

2 quarts organic or homemade chicken stock

1 tablespoon low-sodium soy sauce

2 star anise, whole

2 tablespoons fresh ginger, peeled and chopped

1 tablespoon garlic, peeled and chopped

1 teaspoon cumin seeds

1 teaspoon fennel seeds

1 bunch basil

one 4-pound chicken, cleaned and quartered

MOJO (SAUCE)

2 tablespoons peanut oil

4 cloves garlic, peeled and sliced thin

1 tablespoon scallions, white part only, sliced thin

1 tablespoon fresh ginger, peeled and minced

1 tablespoon low-sodium soy sauce

1 tablespoon sherry vinegar

½ cup fresh cilantro, coarsely chopped, for garnish

To prepare the roast calabaza, preheat the oven to 350°F. Mix the oil, brown sugar, cinnamon, and vanilla together. Coat the calabaza with the mixture and place on a sheet pan. Cover with foil and bake until the calabaza becomes tender, about 30 minutes. Uncover the pan and mix in the corn. Cook uncovered for 10 minutes. Mix in the cilantro and parsley. Season to taste, with salt and pepper. Set aside.

In a large soup or stock pot, combine the stock, soy sauce, star anise, ginger, garlic, cumin seeds, fennel seeds, and basil over medium-high heat. Bring to a boil, reduce to a simmer, and add the chicken. Cook until cooked through, about 35 to 45 minutes. Using tongs, transfer the chicken pieces to a serving plate.

For the mojo, heat the peanut oil in a sauté pan. When the oil is smoking, quickly remove the pan from the heat and add the garlic, scallions, ginger, soy sauce, and vinegar, shaking the pan so nothing burns.

To serve, spread the roast calabaza and corn on a serving plate. Top with the chicken pieces, and pour the sizzling oil over the chicken. Sprinkle the cilantro on top and serve immediately.

The calabaza—which is literally Spanish for pumpkin, one of the foods in the powerfood categories—is popular throughout the Caribbean as well as South and Central America. Also called West Indian pumpkin, calabazas are round in shape and can range in size from as small as a canteloupe to as large as a watermelon. Its skin color can range from green to pale tan to light red orange. Its firm and succulent flesh is bright orange, and it has a sweet flavor, not unlike that of butternut squash. It can be found year-round in Latin markets and large supermarkets.

Nutritional information per 1-person serving:

	Serving	Calories	Total Fat	Carbs.	Fiber	Sugars	Protein	Antioxidant Rating
Star Anise and Ginger Chicken in Mojo	**6 ounces**	**321**	**10.6g**	**0**	**0**	**0**	**52.9g**	**1**
Calabaza and Corn	1 cup	147	5.5g	30g	3g	8g	3.5g	2

Shrimp with a Mango-Ginger Sauce—Dinner

CHEF: XIOMARA ARDOLINA   SERVES 2

LATIN
POWER-
FOODS

Chef Xiomara Ardolina enjoys great depth of flavor—as you can see here—combined with a variety of ingredients. She recommends serving this dish with a mash of malanga, a delicious nut-flavored tuber, but you can serve it on its own, with a green leafy salad, and/or with your favorite mashed potatoes (though that will make it a bit heavier . . .). This recipe contains the Latin powerfood garlic, and bell peppers, onions, shrimp, and chayote.

MANGO-GINGER SAUCE

1 teaspoon plus ½ cup canola oil

2 shallots, peeled and finely diced

1 red bell pepper, seeded and diced

1 tablespoon fresh ginger, minced

1 tablespoon garlic, peeled and minced

2 mangoes, peeled, seeded, and chopped

½ cup Chinese rice cooking wine

½ cup dark rum

salt and pepper to taste

SOYBEAN SAUCE

1 teaspoon canola oil

2 shallots, peeled and finely diced

1 tablespoon fresh ginger, peeled and minced

1 tablespoon garlic, peeled and minced

½ cup white wine

¼ cup Chinese rice cooking wine

¼ cup dark balsamic vinegar

1½ tablespoons soybean paste (available in Asian markets)

½ cup fresh orange juice

½ pound unsalted butter, melted

VEGETABLES

1 teaspoon canola (or olive) oil

2 tablespoons white onions, sliced

2 tablespoons red bell peppers, chopped

2 tablespoons yellow bell peppers, chopped

1 baby bok choy, cut lengthwise into 4 pieces

¼ cup carrots, julienned

¼ cup chayote, julienned (Mexican squash, available in Latin markets, large supermarkets, and online)

¼ cup Napa cabbage, sliced

salt and pepper to taste

SHRIMP

1 teaspoon canola (or olive) oil

10 jumbo (tiger) shrimp, peeled and deveined

1 teaspoon garlic, peeled and minced

¼ cup white wine

1 tablespoon Mango-Ginger Sauce

To make the Mango-Ginger Sauce, heat 1 teaspoon of oil in a medium frying pan over medium-high heat. Sauté the shallots and pepper with ginger and garlic. Add the mango, and then add the rice wine and rum and cook until the mango softens, about 5 minutes. Transfer to a food processor and blend as you slowly add the remaining ½ cup of oil. Add salt and pepper and set aside.

To make the Soybean Sauce, heat 1 teaspoon of oil in a medium frying pan over medium-high heat. Sauté the shallots, ginger, and garlic. Add the white wine and rice wine, balsamic vinegar, soybean paste, and orange juice, and cook over moderate heat until the liquid is reduced by about half, approximately 15 minutes. Then, as you whisk, slowly add the butter. Set aside.

Next, heat the oil in a medium frying pan over medium heat. Add the onions, bell peppers, bok choy, carrots, chayote, cabbage, and salt and pepper. Sauté until the vegetables start to soften (but are still crisp; don't overcook), 5 to 8 minutes. Set aside.

Finally, to prepare the shrimp, heat the canola oil in a medium frying pan over medium-high heat. Sauté the shrimp with garlic and white wine and cook until the shrimp starts to turn pink, about 3 minutes. Add the Mango-Ginger Sauce; make sure the shrimp is well coated.

To serve, use a serving platter or evenly distribute the shrimp and sautéed vegetables onto two plates. Drizzle a quarter cup of the Soybean Sauce on top and serve.

Nutritional information per 1-person serving:

	Serving	Calories	Total Fat	Carbs.	Fiber	Sugars	Protein	Antioxidant Rating
6 ounces shrimp with 1 tablespoon Mango Sauce and ¹/₄ cup Soybean Sauce and side of vegetables		241	14g	6g	6g	9g	12.4g	2
Mango Sauce	1 table-spoon	111	7g	5g	6g	4g	0.5g	2
Soybean Sauce	¹/₄ cup	373	37g	4.2g	0	4g	0.2g	1
Malanga	1 cup	132	0.5g	32g	2g	30g	2g	3
Green Salad	2 cups	46	0	9g	4g	0	3g	2

*F*ruit with Chile de Árbol and Lime Juice—Snack

CHEF: SUE TORRES   SERVES 6

● ●

LATIN
POWER-
FOODS

*This gorgeous, tasty, and slightly sparky snack is guaranteed to bright-
en even the cloudiest of days! Why not make some to serve for brunch
on Sunday, and then take to work on Monday? (That is, of course, if
you've got any left over. . . .) Chile de árbol is one of my Latin powerfoods, and pineapple and lime are in the powerfood categories.*

2 cups watermelon, cut into 1-inch cubes
and seeded

2 cups golden pineapple, cored, cut into
1-inch cubes

2 cups cantaloupe, cut into 1-inch cubes

2 cups honeydew, cut into 1-inch cubes

2 limes, cut into wedges (for squeezing)

2 tablespoons chile de árbol powder
(found in large supermarkets, Latin
markets, or online)

salt to taste

Combine the fruit in a large bowl. Squeeze the lime juice over the fruit.
Sprinkle with chile powder and a little salt. Serve immediately.

Nutritional information per 1-person serving:

	Serving	Calories	Total Fat	Carbs.	Fiber	Sugars	Protein	Antioxidant Rating
Fruit with chile de árbol and lime juice	1 cup	120	0	29.7g	1.6g	15.3g	1.6g	3

*T*oasted Garbanzo Beans—Snack

CHEF: ARLEN GARGAGLIANO   SERVES 4

● ●

LATIN POWER-FOODS

This super-easy and super-tasty snack is healthy and portable! You can always turn the heat higher—or lower—depending on how spicy you like your treats. This snack has two of my Latin powerfoods: garbanzos and chile (in the form of chili powder). Lime is in one of the powerfood categories.

one 15.5-ounce can garbanzos (chickpeas)   ½ teaspoon chili powder or to taste

2 tablespoons olive oil   ½ teaspoon coarse sea salt or to taste

½ teaspoon ground cumin or to taste   1 lime wedge

Preheat the oven to 450°F. Drain and rinse the can of garbanzos. Blot them dry with a paper towel. In a bowl, toss the beans with the olive oil, and ¼ teaspoon each of the cumin, chili powder, and salt. Spread on a baking sheet, and bake for about 35 minutes, until toasted and crunchy. Check frequently, using a spatula to move the beans around. As it gets toward the end of the cooking time, watch the beans carefully to avoid burning. Once they're done, let them cool for about 5 minutes, and then transfer them to a small ceramic serving dish (like Spanish-style terra-cotta dishes) and add the remaining cumin, chili powder, and sea salt and serve. If you're not serving them at that moment, let them cool completely, and store in an airtight container for up to one week. Squeeze the juice from the lime wedge on top of the beans just before serving.

Nutritional information per 1-person serving:

	Serving	Calories	Total Fat	Carbs.	Fiber	Sugars	Protein	Antioxidant Rating
Toasted Garbanzo Beans	½ cup	143	1.4g	27.1g	5.3g	0	5.9g	2

*C*ucumber Raita with Coconut—Snack

CHEF: ARLEN GARGAGLIANO   SERVES 8

● ●

LATIN
POWER-
FOODS

This cooling saladlike dish—an interpretation of an Indian treat that made its way to the Caribbean—is one that my coauthor enjoys as an afternoon snack, alongside a spicy meal, or even by itself for breakfast. The cayenne or chile pepper adds a nice kick—but you can always leave that out. Chile pepper is one of my Latin powerfoods.

1 ½ cups plain low-fat yogurt

2 ounces light coconut milk

cayenne or chile pepper, to taste

½ cup fresh mint leaves, coarsely chopped

3 cucumbers, peeled, seeded, and cut into ¼-inch cubes

2 tablespoons shredded coconut, optional (I like the sweetened kind, but either one is fine)

*I*n a medium bowl, combine the yogurt and coconut milk. Add the pepper. Stir in the mint. Add the cucumbers. Cover and refrigerate for at least an hour (and up to 2 days). Sprinkle coconut flakes on top just before serving.

Nutritional information per 1-person serving:

	Serving	Calories	Total Fat	Carbs.	Fiber	Sugars	Protein	Antioxidant Rating
Cucumber-Coconut Raita with shredded coconut	½ cup	74.5	4.6g	5.9g	1.2g	4.4g	3.3g	I

Note: Enjoy the shredded coconut with this—it will only add 20 calories and 2 grams of fat; no need to take it out unless you like it better that way.

TRACK ONE: RECAP

You should've decreased your body fat between two and four percent and lost about four to six pounds in the first two weeks. By eating the seven Latin powerfoods and incorporating snacks into your daily meal plan, your metabolism is working much more efficiently and your body is flushing out the toxins in your cells. Because you're eating a more well-balanced and regular diet, you should feel lighter and more positive, and cravings you may have had before—mainly for carbs and high-fat foods—should be greatly lessened. The effects on your body will pick up even more momentum in the next track, allowing you to reach a level where it will be second nature to regulate your caloric intake and thus maintain your bombshell body.

Keep in mind that for everyone—those who see scale differences and those who don't—the Hot Latin Diet will be a huge step toward better health. Drinking lots of water will speed up the detoxing process.

The next step, Track Two, will bring you even more rewards—both in terms of how you feel and how you look!

Track Two: The Next Four Weeks

So now you know the deal, right? You've got a repertoire of recipes and you're eating your seven Latin powerfoods, you've gotten your exercise routine, and you're ready to keep moving forward. (For exercise tips, see the guidelines starting on p. 177.) The next step is here! I'm adding just a few more recipes to your repertoire—which you'll see in a moment. These dishes, as I've mentioned, incorporate some additional ingredients, and a bit more lean meat for maintenance of strength, muscle mass, power, and stamina. You'll also notice that our focus in this phase has turned to the wonders of garbanzo beans. Whether in Xiomara's tasty salad or in Michelle Bernstein's Spiced-up Hummus, we want you to think garbanzos. Their high fiber content and low fat and sugar levels make them the perfect food to fight cravings and maintain your intestinal flora health.

While our focus in Track One was to rid your body of all the harmful toxins we come to accumulate over the years, Track Two is about keeping up the good work and continuing to lose weight by burning your body's excess fat. Although it may seem that the rapid weight loss of the past two weeks stagnates a bit during this phase, you should expect to lose around one or two pounds a week. The reason for this is that your body has gotten rid of its excess water and is now burning actual fat, which, as we all know, does not happen as quickly. So the good news is while your weight loss may *seem* slower, it is in fact more significant and long-lasting. Don't forget—you should also bring in the dishes you were enjoying from Track One and mix and match; while these dishes are slightly higher in calories (you will be consuming between 1,800 and 2,000 calories a day), they are totally interchangeable.

INTRODUCING YOUR OWN VARIATIONS

The recipes listed for enjoying after the first two weeks include some richer ingredients and more protein for maintenance of strength, muscle mass, power, and stamina. Again, all of the recipes in the Hot Latin Diet are for you to prepare and experiment with; you can mix some ingredients around, or eat the same ones a couple of times a week, so as to gain familiarity with their preparation. Remember, take it one step at a time—but start stepping!

As we've discussed, the nice thing about this fabulous collection of recipes is their ability to be varied. Let me tell you my own variation on one of them: one of my favorite treats in this book is chef Sue Torres's Cilantro Pesto, which she suggests serving atop grilled veggies. Now this pesto—made with two (cilantro and garlic) of our seven Latin powerfoods, not to mention pine nuts—can be varied and served in many ways. For example, I was craving this pesto not too long ago, but I didn't have pine nuts on hand—but I did have pecans. So I toasted the pecans and incorporated them the way Sue had suggested.

So keep this openness in mind as you work on making these recipes your own—and vary them depending on what you like, what you have on hand, and what you'd like to try, though do keep an eye out for your caloric intake!

In creating your own variations on the recipes for Track Two, here are a few things you need to keep in mind for each meal of the day.

BREAKFAST

As in Track One, breakfast is the time to eat those high-protein foods and carbs, because you'll need them to power through your day. You'll even find *torrejas* (Spanish French toast) on your list of recipes for this phase! By preparing the *torrejas* with whole-grain bread instead of your regular white loaf or baguette, chef Daisy Martínez makes this morning treat into a healthy delight that's low on the calories. So I suggest you think of some of your favorite breakfast dishes, and think about replacing the traditional ingredients with their healthy, wholesome counterparts.

LUNCH

No matter how hectic your day may be, it's important that you never— and mark my words—ever skip lunch. Unfortunately, the fast pace of modern life can sometimes make it difficult to sit down to a healthy lunch, let alone have the time to cook an entire meal. If you don't have time to cook the delicious salmon or Coriander-Crusted Chicken recipes you will find below, what I suggest you do is fix yourself a quick salad with similar ingredients. Chicken, turkey, avocado, and tomatoes are a few fantastic ingredients you can combine for a quick and satisfying meal that will not send you off track.

DINNER

For dinner, continue to eat meals low in carbs, although in Track Two you should feel free to eat as many vegetables as possible. Not only will these give you the minerals and vitamins you need, but they will contribute to keeping your intestinal flora healthy—a key factor in the elimination of all the toxins in your body.

Remember, these six dishes (plus our three new snacks) are all—once again—easily adaptable, and great fun to make, serve, and, of course, eat! Like those from Track One, they incorporate many ingredients that may be new to you. Keep that positive outlook going—and your palate open and ready. *¡Buen provecho!* Enjoy!

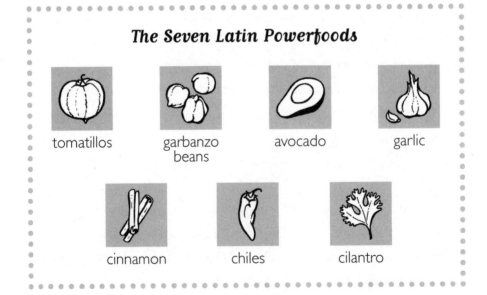

The Seven Latin Powerfoods

tomatillos   garbanzo beans   avocado   garlic

cinnamon   chiles   cilantro

Ejotes con Huevo (Fresh String Beans with Egg)— Breakfast

CHEF: ZARELA MARTÍNEZ

● ●

LATIN POWER-FOODS

This dish, from Zarela's childhood in Mexico, could be a breakfast or a side dish—and it's very flexible: vegetarians can make it without the eggs, and other vegetables can be substituted for the string beans. Also, Pico de Gallo, a typical Mexican-style salsa, makes about 4 cups, so you can use it atop grilled veggies, chicken, meat, or fish—or with chips. Chef Martínez's prep tip: the beans must be tossed very quickly with the sauce and egg, almost as if you were stir-frying. This recipe is packed with three of my Latin powerfoods—chiles, garlic, and cilantro—as well as tomatoes, lime, and egg. This is a great dish for breakfast or lunch.

PICO DE GALLO

2 to 4 fresh chiles, either jalapeño or serrano, or to taste, tops removed but not seeded, finely chopped

1 garlic clove, peeled and minced

4 large ripe red tomatoes, about 2 ½ pounds, peeled but not seeded, and coarsely chopped

6 to 8 scallions, both light and dark green parts, finely chopped

¼ cup (loosely packed) fresh cilantro leaves, finely chopped

1 teaspoon dried Mexican oregano (available in Latin markets or online) or to taste, crumbled

juice of 1 large lime

salt to taste

BEANS

1 pound string beans, trimmed, strings removed if necessary, cut into 1-inch pieces

2 tablespoons vegetable oil

1 cup Pico de Gallo Norteño

1 egg

pepper to taste

*T*o make the Pico de Gallo, place all the ingredients in a large bowl, but be sure to add the chiles a little at a time, tasting until it's as hot as you'd like it. If the tomatoes aren't too juicy, add about ½ cup of cold water to the mix so that the mixture reaches a light salsa consistency. Stir to mix. Add the salt to taste. Use immediately, or cover and refrigerate for up 1 day.

In a large pot of rapidly boiling water, blanch the beans until slightly tender but still crunchy, about 2 minutes. Drain thoroughly.

In a large skillet, heat the oil over high heat until hot and bubbling. Add 1 cup of the Pico de Gallo and sauté until liquid is nearly evaporated, about 2 minutes. Add the drained beans and cook, tossing rapidly until the beans start to soften, about 1½ to 2 minutes.

Beat the egg and strain through a strainer into a small bowl. Add to the bean mixture and cook, tossing and stirring, just until egg is set, a minute or less. Season to taste with salt and pepper and serve immediately.

Nutritional information per 1-person serving:

	Serving	Calories	Total Fat	Carbs.	Fiber	Sugars	Protein	Antioxidant Rating
1 cup Pico de Gallo & 1 cup Ejotes con Huevo		225	17g	16g	7.8g	1.6g	7.5g	3
Pico de Gallo	1 cup	40	0	8g	4g	0	4g	3
Ejotes con Huevo	1 cup	185	17g	8g	3.8g	1.6g	3.5g	1
Ejotes sin Huevo	1 cup	150	14g	8g	3.8g	1.6g	1g	1

Torrejas

CHEF: DAISY MARTÍNEZ

SERVES 4

LATIN
POWER-
FOODS

This Latin-style French toast, called torrejas in Spain, is—as chef Daisy Martínez says—an ingenious way for a homemaker to make use of stale bread. Daisy says that she enjoys both the sweet (listed here) and savory versions (think side dish) and has enjoyed both immensely. The sugar in this recipe is optional; the cinnamon and extracts add tons of flavor. Daisy recommends using day-old Cuban bread, but I'd like to suggest brown or whole-grain bread as a more nutritional choice. This dish has eggs, as well as one of the top seasonings (and a Latin powerfood): cinnamon.

eight 1-inch slices of crusty day-old brown or whole-grain bread

5 jumbo organic eggs, beaten

1 cup organic 2% milk

⅛ teaspoon almond extract

½ teaspoon vanilla extract

canola oil spray

3 tablespoons turbinado sugar (optional)

¼ teaspoon ground cinnamon

Set the bread in a casserole large enough to accommodate it comfortably. In a bowl, mix the eggs, milk, and extracts together and pour them over the bread, allowing it to soak completely. Flip the bread over when one side appears to be saturated.

Spray a skillet liberally with oil spray and heat over medium-high heat. Place the bread slices in the skillet, lower the heat to low, and cook until golden brown and firm on the bottom, between 3 and 5 minutes. Flip and cook the other side until golden on the bottom, another 3 to 5 minutes. Remove and set on serving platter.

Mix the sugar and cinnamon together, and dust the *torrejas* on the platter. Serve warm, with your favorite fruit compote or preserves.

	Serving	Calories	Total Fat	Carbs.	Fiber	Sugars	Protein	Antioxidant Rating
Torrejas with sugar or preserves	2 slices	338	10g	39g	5g	15g	14.9g	1
Torrejas	2 slices	292	10g	27g	5g	3g	14.9g	1
Sugar or preserves	1 table-spoon	46	0	12g	0	12g	0	1

Grilled Salmon with Green Sauce and Tomatillo-Pineapple Salsa—Lunch

CHEF: SUE TORRES

● ●

LATIN POWER-FOODS

If you're a salmon fan, this recipe is definitely for you! Actually, even if you're not, this one may sway you. Here the fleshy fish is beautifully balanced—in both color and flavor—by both wonderful sauces. And, if you've never used tomatillos before, this is a perfect introduction to this typical Mexican tomato-like veggie. Actually, the individual components of this dish, which could be for lunch or dinner, are easily adaptable to other recipes. This recipe is packed with several Latin powerfoods: tomatillos, chiles, avocados, and cilantro. It also has lime, jícama, onion, and pineapple.

GREEN SAUCE

3/4 cup water

2 tomatillos, coarsely chopped (about 1 cup)

2 serrano chiles, stemmed but not seeded, coarsely chopped

1 1/2 avocados, preferably Mexican Hass, peeled and seeded (about 1 cup packed)

1 tablespoon salt

juice of 1 lime (about 1/8 cup)

1/4 cup fresh cilantro, chopped (optional)

TOMATILLO-PINEAPPLE SALSA

3/4 cup jícama, cut into 1/4-inch dice

1/2 cup red onion, cut into 1/4-inch dice

1/2 cup pineapple, cut into 1/4-inch dice

1 cup tomatillos, cut into 1/4-inch dice

2 tablespoons fresh cilantro (leaves and stems), coarsely chopped

juice of 1 lime (about 1/8 cup)

1/8 of an habanero chile, seeded and finely minced

1 teaspoon salt

1/2 teaspoon pepper

1/8 cup sunflower (or your favorite) oil

SALMON

four 6-ounce wild salmon fillets, with skin   1 tablespoon oil

salt and pepper   4 lime wedges

*T*o make the Green Sauce, pour the water into the bottom of a blender. Add the tomatillos and serranos and blend until puréed. Add the avocado, salt, and lime (and cilantro, if desired). Mix until well blended. Set aside, or cover and refrigerate for up to 3 hours.

In a medium-size bowl, combine the jícama, red onion, and pineapple, and tomatillos. Stir in the cilantro, lime juice, habanero, salt, and pepper. Add the oil and stir until well coated. Let sit for an hour at room temperature and correct seasoning, or cover and refrigerate for up to 3 days.

Season salmon fillets with salt and pepper. Heat oil in a medium-size stainless steel saucepan over a medium-high flame until hot but not smoking. Add 4 fillets, skin side down, and sear until the skin is well browned, about 4 minutes. Turn fillets over and sear until just cooked through, 3 to 4 minutes more. Transfer to serving platter and keep warm. (You also have the option to grill the salmon.)

Set four plates up for serving, and ladle about two ounces of the Green Sauce into each plate. Add 1 heaping tablespoon of the salsa, add a salmon fillet, and top with a teaspoon of the fruit salsa. Garnish with a fresh lime wedge, and serve.

Nutritional information per 1-person serving:

	Serving	Calories	Total Fat	Carbs.	Fiber	Sugars	Protein	Antioxidant Rating
Salmon with both sauces		529	30.8g	10.3g	8.2g	8.8g	45.3g	3
Grilled Salmon	6 ounces	349	17.8g	0	0	0	43.2g	1
Green Sauce	½ cup	103	8.3g	5.5g	4.4g	0.9g	1.5g	3
Tomatillo-Pineapple Sauce	1 cup	77	4.7g	4.8g	3.8g	7.9g	0.6g	2

Coriander-Crusted Chicken Breast with Grilled Chipotle-Sparked Potatoes and Mustard Greens—Dinner

CHEF: SUE TORRES

SERVES 4 TO 6

● ●

LATIN POWER-FOODS

The nice part about this Coriander-Crusted Chicken—aside from the incredible flavor—is the texture: the ground seeds become a delicious crust that contrasts beautifully with the tender chicken meat. And, true to chef Sue Torres's devotion to contrast in flavor and color, this dish makes a wonderful presentation of both. And, if you've got any chicken left over, it's great in a sandwich on fresh Italian bread, with this same chef's wonderful Cilantro Pesto (page 148), and a few slices of tomato. Of course, the grilled potatoes are great, too! This recipe has two Latin powerfoods: chiles (chipotle) and garlic. It also has chicken and mustard greens (or spinach).

POTATOES

1 tablespoon unsalted butter

2 tablespoons chipotle purée (from a 7-ounce can of chipotle peppers in adobo sauce, puréed in a blender or food processor)

6 Yukon Gold (or red bliss) potatoes, scrubbed and sliced ¼ inch thick

3 tablespoons olive oil

CHICKEN

kosher or sea salt and pepper

6 free-range chicken breast halves, about 3 pounds

¼ cup coriander seeds, freshly ground (a coffee grinder is perfect for this)

sunflower or canola oil, enough to coat the pan

GREENS

2 bunches mustard greens (about 1½ pounds), stems and center ribs discarded, leaves halved (you can also use fresh spinach)

¼ cup olive oil

2 garlic cloves, minced

½ cup water

½ teaspoon salt or to taste

*T*o prepare the potatoes, heat a grill to medium high. Melt the butter, then combine it in a bowl with the chipotle purée. Place the potatoes on a sheet pan, and brush both sides with the olive oil. Grill the potatoes until tender, about 5 minutes on each side. As soon as they're done, put them in a bowl with the chipotle mixture, and stir until well blended. Cover and set aside. As soon as they're cool enough to handle, cut them into ¼-inch dice. (Note: you can also broil the potatoes, with a bit of oil, and then use the chipotle mixture as directed.)

To prepare the chicken, sprinkle salt and pepper on each of the chicken breast halves. Spread the ground coriander on a plate. Evenly coat breast halves on both sides. Heat a medium-size sauté pan over moderately high heat. Add the oil and heat until hot, but not smoking. Add the chicken pieces and sear, for about 4 minutes per side. Lower the heat, and continue cooking until nicely brown on the outside, and no longer pink in the center, about 20 minutes. Cover with foil to keep warm while you prepare the mustard greens.

Note: If you're using mustard greens, blanch them for two minutes in rapidly boiling salted water, and then place them immediately in an ice bath. If you're using spinach—or after blanching the mustard greens—heat a medium-size sauté pan over moderately high heat. Add oil and heat until hot, but not smoking. Add the garlic and stir. Add half the greens and toss with tongs to coat with oil, adding remaining half as greens wilt. Add water and salt. Cover and cook, stirring occasionally, until the greens are just tender and most of the liquid is evaporated, about 5 minutes. Taste and season as desired.

To serve, start with the potatoes in the middle of the plate; then lay the greens at the bottom (like a kind of smiley face). Sue likes to then cut the chicken breasts into 1/4-inch-thick slices, and place them on the plate in a semicircle partially on the mustard greens so they have a little height and depth.

Nutritional information per 1-person serving:

	Serving	Calories	Total Fat	Carbs.	Fiber	Sugars	Protein	Antioxidant Rating
6 ounces chicken with with 1/2 cup greens and 1 cup potatoes		600.5	24.2g	37g	3.8g	39g	57.7g	4
Chipotle-Sparked Potatoes	1 cup	222	8.5g	34.6g	2.4g	2.6g	3g	4
Mustard Greens or Spinach	1/2 cup	97.5	9.6g	2.4g	1.5g	0.3g	1.8g	3

*P*an-Seared Red Snapper with Grapefruit-Avocado Salsa—Dinner

CHEF: DAISY MARTÍNEZ   SERVES 4

● ●

LATIN POWER-FOODS

Perfect for a steamy summer day—or to bring in flavors of summer on a wintry day—this dish, with the balance of a citrus and avocado salsa, works beautifully with the tender flavor of the snapper. Daisy, whose culinary influences stem in great part from her Puerto Rican abuelitos (grandparents), likes to serve this dish with yellow rice or a green leafy salad. Avocados and cilantro are the two Latin powerfoods in this recipe. onion and snapper are in the powerfood categories.

2 large grapefruit, sectioned

1 small red onion, diced

1 jalapeño pepper, seeded and chopped

1 teaspoon olive oil

1 lemon, juiced

four 6-ounce red snapper fillets

salt and fresh ground pepper

1 teaspoon canola oil

2 Hass avocados, peeled, seeded, and cut into ¼-inch dice

¼ cup fresh cilantro leaves, chopped

Dice the grapefruit sections, and toss with the diced red onion and jalapeño. Drizzle with olive oil and lemon juice, and set aside in the fridge.

Season the fillets with salt and pepper. Brush the bottom of a non-stick skillet with the canola oil, and set over medium-high heat. Place the fillets, skin side down, into the pan, and cook until the skin is crispy, between 3 and 4 minutes. Flip the fish over and cook until the fish can flake, another 1 to 2 minutes.

Pull your salsa out of the fridge, add the avocado and cilantro, toss, and check the seasoning. Use a ladle to put about 2 ounces of sauce on each serving plate. Place the fillet on top and serve.

Nutritional information per 1-person serving:

	Serving	Calories	Total Fat	Carbs.	Fiber	Sugars	Protein	Antioxidant Rating
6 ounces Snapper with 1 cup Salsa		301	13.5g	14.6g	5.6g	8.2g	32g	3
Pan-Seared Red Snapper	6 ounces	152	2.7g	0	0	0	30g	1
Grapefruit-Avocado Salsa	1 cup	149	10.8g	14.6g	5.6g	8.2g	2g	3
Yellow Rice	1 cup	190	0	43g	0.5g	0.5g	4g	1
Green Salad	1 cup	46	0	9g	4g	0	3g	2

Xiomara Salad—Dinner

CHEF: XIOMARA ARDOLINA   SERVES 2

● ●

LATIN
POWER-
FOODS

This gorgeous and tasty salad can easily be adapted for the non-meat-eater—by marinating cooked chickpeas for about half an hour (or more!) in Xiomara's wonderful Cuban-style marinade. If you are using turkey, though, you'll have to start the day before. This recipe contains two of my Latin powerfoods: garlic and avocado. It also has lime, turkey, onions, radish, and tomatoes.

MARINADE

2 cups fresh orange juice

2 cups fresh lime juice

1 tablespoon oregano

1 tablespoon garlic, chopped

2 bay leaves

salt and pepper to taste

1 whole (about 12 ounces) free-range turkey breast

SALAD

2 handfuls baby mixed greens

2 handfuls baby yellow (or regular green) frisée

¼ cup red onions, thinly sliced

¼ cup cucumbers (hot house), sliced

¼ cup radish, thinly sliced

8 pear tomatoes, halved

1½ tablespoons fresh lemon juice

1½ tablespoons olive oil

½ cup avocado, cubed

salt and freshly ground black pepper to taste

½ cup cooked chickpeas

*T*o prepare the marinade, whisk the orange juice, lime juice, oregano, and garlic together. Stir in the bay leaves. Taste and season with salt and pepper. Pour over the turkey breast. Store in a sealed container overnight in the refrigerator.

Preheat the oven to 350°F. Place the turkey breast, with the marinade, in an ovenproof casserole. Bake uncovered, basting every 20 minutes, until cooked through, about 45 minutes (be careful not to overcook). Cool and add to the salad (see below), or cover and chill in the refrigerator for up to 2 days.

Cut the turkey breast halves into bite-size chunks. Combine them with the greens, frisée, onions, cucumbers, radish, and tomatoes. Stir in the lemon juice and olive oil. Add the avocado and salt and pepper, and garnish the salad with the chickpeas. Serve immediately.

Nutritional information per 1-person serving:

	Serving	Calories	Total Fat	Carbs.	Fiber	Sugars	Protein	Antioxidant Rating
Xiomara Salad with 6 ounces turkey and 1/8 cup crumbled cheese on top		550	30.4g	11.6g	11.4g	0.8g	59.4g	1
Xiomara Salad with 1 cup chickpeas, no cheese		470	19.6g	64.1g	18.3g	0.8g	14.2g	1
1/8 cup gorgonzola or cabrales		98	8g	1.8g	0.4g	0	6.2g	1

Spiced-Up Hummus—Snack

CHEF: MICHELLE BERNSTEIN

LATIN POWER-FOODS

This supersimple, nicely spiced and energy-packed snack is easy to prepare, store, and bring to work in a small container! Though this snack is Middle Eastern in origin, chef Michelle Bernstein serves it to complement many of her Latin dishes. She recommends enjoying with fresh carrot sticks or baked pita chips. This snack has the Latin powerfoods garbanzo beans and garlic.

one 14-ounce can of chickpeas, rinsed and drained

1 clove garlic, peeled and coarsely chopped

¼ cup fresh-squeezed lemon juice

½ cup tahini paste

1 teaspoon cayenne pepper

¼ teaspoon ground ginger

¼ teaspoon ground cumin

¼ cup water

2 tablespoon extra-virgin olive oil

1 cup scallions, white and light green parts, sliced thin

kosher salt and freshly ground black pepper to taste

Combine the chickpeas, garlic, lemon juice, tahini paste, and spices in a food processor fitted with the metal blade. Add the water and oil, and process until smooth. Fold in the scallions and season with salt and pepper. Refrigerate in an airtight container for at least an hour to chill, and up to 5 days.

Nutritional information per 1-person serving:

	Serving	Calories	Total Fat	Carbs.	Fiber	Sugars	Protein	Antioxidant Rating
½ cup Spiced-Up Hummus		218	10.6g	24.7g	4.9g	0.6g	6g	1
carrots	1 cup	52	0	12.3g	3.5g	5.8g	1.2g	3
pita chips	1 cup	130	5g	19g	2g	0.5g	3g	1

$\mathcal{E}$spinacas (Wilted Spinach)—Snack

CHEF: ZARELA MARTÍNEZ   SERVES 2 TO 4

● ●

LATIN POWER-FOODS

In chef Zarela Martínez's childhood, she enjoyed these leafy greens, called quelites (which is the Mexican name for sautéed greens). This very simple, light, and delicious jalapeño-sparked vegetable dish makes a great afternoon snack—or a wonderful side dish. You can also add cooked beans (black, garbanzo, or your favorite) and easily expand this side dish into a meal. This snack has two Latin powerfoods: jalapeño pepper and cilantro. It also has tomato and spinach.

2 to 3 tablespoons vegetable oil

1 medium tomato, coarsely chopped

3 scallions, white and light green parts, finely chopped

1 clove garlic, peeled and minced

1 jalapeño pepper, or more to taste, seeded if desired, finely chopped

2 tablespoons fresh cilantro, chopped

1 bunch spinach (about 2 cups packed or a 10-ounce package), well rinsed and stemmed

salt to taste

*I*n a large wide skillet, heat oil over high heat until a drop of water sputters on contact. Add the chopped tomato, scallions, garlic, jalapeño, and cilantro. Sauté rapidly for about 30 seconds. Add the spinach in large handfuls, stirring to distribute. Cook spinach, uncovered, just until wilted, about 3 minutes. Add salt to taste and serve at once.

Nutritional information per 1-person serving:

	Serving	Calories	Total Fat	Carbs.	Fiber	Sugars	Protein	Antioxidant Rating
Espinacas	1 cup	160	11g	8g	6g	2g	4g	3
1 cup Espinacas with 1 cup black beans		379	12.5g	45.1g	21.8g	2g	18g	4

Soursop-Mango Blush Batida (Shake)—Snack

CHEF: DAISY MARTÍNEZ   SERVES 2 TO 4 (MAKES ABOUT 4 CUPS)

● ●

Batidas—shakes—come in many forms throughout the Americas. This one combines the tropical flavors of soursop and mango, with our old familiar—and just as lovely—strawberries. Chef Daisy Martínez's choice is guaranteed to leave you with a sweet taste in your mouth, and a bounce in your step! Mango is in one of the Latin powerfood categories.

½ cup crushed ice

1 ½ cups or one 12-ounce can of soursop (guanabana) nectar (available in Latin markets, larger supermarkets, or online)

2 scoops mango sorbet

½ cup evaporated skim milk

4 strawberries, hulls removed

Combine the crushed ice and nectar in a blender and pulse several times. Add the sorbet, milk, and strawberries and blend completely. Serve immediately in tall glasses. (You can chill the glasses before serving!)

Nutritional information per 1-person serving:

	Serving	Calories	Total Fat	Carbs.	Fiber	Sugars	Protein	Antioxidant Rating
Soursop-Mango Blush Batida	1 cup	230	1g	72g	2g	70g	0	2

TRACK TWO RECAP

At this point, you should be feeling—and looking—significantly better than you did just six weeks ago. You've probably lost between twelve and eighteen pounds so far and decreased your body fat by between 8 and 10 percent, so you should be feeling much lighter and very accomplished. Mentally you should feel confident because your change in lifestyle, which was a conscious decision that required some major changes, has proven to be well worth it.

What about the future? Well, if the Hot Latin Diet has helped you achieve your ideal weight and size, you should continue to stay on it. Keep eating those Latin powerfoods! And do read my tips in the next section for how to maintain your weight. If you still have many pounds to shed, you should stay on Track Two (using the recipes in both Track One and Track Two, as well as the ones you've created yourself using the seven Latin powerfoods) until you reach your desired weight. Also, increase your physical activity to between thirty and ninety minutes, at least three times a week. This movement, along with this diet, will help you to lose more pounds. I'd also suggest going to get a physical. It's important to get your numbers checked so you can see, physiologically speaking, where you are. This will also help you address the question of how many more pounds you might want to lose.

Remember, don't beat yourself up if from time to time you break down and have, say, that slice of chocolate cake at your nephew's birthday party. Just let it go and jump right back on track—and stay focused until you achieve that healthier, slimmer body you've been dreaming of. You and I both know you can do it!

Track Three: Week Seven and Beyond

By the time you complete Tracks One and Two, you should be looking several pounds lighter and feeling quite proud of all your accomplishments. But you're not quite done yet. In order to keep the weight off, you need to continue on to Track Three, what I like to call the stabilizing phase.

While Tracks One and Two were all about the weight loss, Track Three is about continuing with the healthy lifestyle you have learned over the course of the past six weeks, and making it second nature. You will find that the recipes contained in Track Three are much more varied and less restrictive. I have even included two dinner recipes with meat—because who wants to live without meat? The key for Track Three is no longer the caloric intake (you will see that it is less restrictive than in the previous two tracks) but the variety of ingredients.

By the time you reach this third and final phase of the diet, you should have met your weight-loss goals—Track Three is about keeping them. Unlike most diets, where when you go off the diet you regain all the weight you've lost, the Hot Latin Diet helps you keep it off by implementing a healthy lifestyle that you will be able to apply for many years to come.

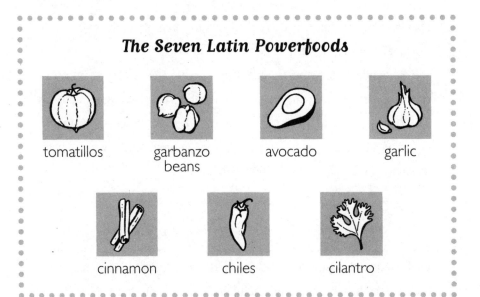

The Seven Latin Powerfoods

tomatillos

garbanzo beans

avocado

garlic

cinnamon

chiles

cilantro

*H*uevos Campesinos (Farmer-Style Eggs) with Red Bell Pepper Sauce—Breakfast

CHEF: XIOMARA ARDOLINA

SERVES 2

● ●

Xiomara's interpretation of a classic Latin American breakfast (which varies depending on where you are—and who's cooking!) combines elements of her native Cuba with a touch of European flair in the form of red bell pepper sauce and Manchego cheese—creating a gorgeous balance of flavor, texture, and color. This breakfast has two Latin power-foods: garlic and culantro (or cilantro). It also has bell peppers, black beans, and onion.

RED BELL PEPPER SAUCE

2 large red bell peppers, roasted, seeded, and skinned, coarsely chopped

2 ounces goat cheese

1 pinch of garlic, minced

4 basil leaves

salt and pepper to taste

1 small whole-wheat flour tortilla

½ cup cooked black beans

½ cup rock shrimp, peeled and deveined

2 teaspoons red bell pepper, diced

2 teaspoons yellow bell pepper, diced

2 teaspoons Spanish onion, diced

1 teaspoon garlic, chopped

1 tablespoon fresh culantro or cilantro, chopped

½ teaspoon unsalted butter

2 eggs, lightly mixed

3 slices Manchego cheese, thinly sliced

*T*o make the Red Bell Pepper Sauce, combine the roasted peppers, goat cheese, garlic, and basil in a blender. Mix until well blended. Season to taste and set aside.

Next, warm the tortilla (you can do this in your tortilla warmer, your toaster oven—or if the tortilla's wrapped in foil, your oven on low heat—or by quickly tossing it in a frying pan). Keep it wrapped in a paper towel or tea towel until you're ready to use it. Warm the black beans in a small saucepan and set them aside.

In a medium frying pan over moderate heat, sauté the rock shrimp with bell peppers, onion, and garlic until the shrimp turn pink and the vegetables start to soften, about 5 minutes. Add the culantro.

To prepare the eggs, melt the butter in a small sauté pan over medium heat. Add the eggs and salt and pepper. Let set for about 30 seconds, and then stir, using a spatula or wooden spoon (depending on how you like your scrambled eggs!). Cook until set, about another 1½ minutes. Remove from heat.

To serve, place the tortilla on a cutting board. Coat it first with a layer of the black beans, then the shrimp with onion and peppers, add the eggs, and cover with slices of Manchego cheese. Use a sharp knife to cut the tortilla in half, and a spatula to set each half on a serving plate. Garnish with the Red Bell Pepper Sauce. Serve immediately.

Nutritional information per 1-person serving:

	Serving	Calories	Total Fat	Carbs.	Fiber	Sugars	Protein	Antioxidant Rating
Huevos and Sauce		422	20.4g	27.6g	12.5g	3.2g	24.8g	3
Red Bell Pepper Sauce		70	4g	7.6g	3.5g	2.7g	3.8g	3
Huevos Campesinos		352	16.4g	20g	9g	0.5g	21g	1

Migas—Mexican-Style Breakfast

CHEF: SUE TORRES

SERVES 4 TO 6

This gorgeous and tasty rendition of a traditional Mexican breakfast is perfect for the first thing in the morning—or brunch. Non-meat-eaters can certainly enjoy this without the chorizo. This dish features two of my Latin powerfoods, chiles (chipotles) and cilantro, as well as tomatoes and eggs.

TOMATO COULIS

2 ½ cups plum or best-available tomatoes, coarsely chopped

½ cup white or Spanish onion (white is most frequently used in Mexico), coarsely chopped

1 tablespoon garlic, coarsely chopped

2 chipotles en adobo (available in cans in Latin markets and large grocery stores)

1 tablespoon salt

1 pinch pepper

4 tablespoons sunflower (or your favorite) oil

2 links Mexican or Spanish chorizo, removed from casing, diced or coarsely chopped

8 eggs, lightly beaten

20 corn tortilla chips, preferably homemade

fresh cilantro for garnish

To make the tomato coulis, place some of the tomato in a blender, and pulse to create a liquidy base. Add the remaining tomato, onion, garlic, chipotles, salt, and pepper. Blend until puréed. Set aside until the rest of the meal is ready (or you can prep it ahead and simply heat the coulis, as described below, just before serving).

To cook the chorizo, heat a medium-size stainless steel saucepan over medium-high heat. Add two tablespoons of oil. Then add the chorizo, and cook, stirring frequently, until the chorizo is golden and cooked through, about 10 minutes. Add the eggs, and when the eggs start to cook, after 1 to 1½ minutes, add the corn chips. Use a wooden spoon to crush the chips as you stir to cook the eggs. Cook until cooked through, about another 3 minutes. Remove from heat.

Heat a medium-size stainless steel saucepan over medium-high heat. Add 2 tablespoons oil. Then add the coulis to "sear" the sauce and bring out the flavors. Stirring frequently, cook until heated through, about five minutes (can be longer if chilled). Set four plates up for serving, and ladle about two ounces of the coulis into each plate. Top with the egg mixture, and a sprinkle of cilantro. Serve immediately.

Nutritional information per 1-person serving:

	Serving	Calories	Total Fat	Carbs.	Fiber	Sugars	Protein	Antioxidant Rating
Eggs, Chorizo, and Coulis as in recipe		565	41g	27.6g	6.3g	0	24.6g	3
Tomato Coulis	1 cup	40	0	8g	4g	0	4g	3
2 Eggs and ½ link Chorizo		525	41g	19.6g	2.3g	0	20.6g	1
2 Eggs without Chorizo		250	26g	10g	1.5g	0	12.2g	1

Quinoa Risotto Primavera—Lunch

CHEF: DAISY MARTÍNEZ

SERVES 4 TO 6

● ●

Daisy's variation on an Italian classic contains a Latin powerfood that dates back to the ancient Incas: quinoa (see more information below). This risotto, which makes a perfect lunch, could also be a side dish—without the turkey sausage—to grilled fish or chicken. This recipe has the Latin powerfood garlic, and quinoa, onion, turkey, and beans.

2 tablespoons olive oil

1 clove garlic, minced

½ cup medium Spanish onion, diced

1½ cups spicy turkey sausage, sliced

1 cup quinoa

1 cup evaporated skim milk

1 cup homemade or organic chicken broth

1 bay leaf

½ cup fava beans

½ cup morel mushrooms, sliced

1 bunch of arugula, washed well, cut into 2-inch pieces

salt and freshly ground black pepper to taste

¼ cup Manchego cheese, shredded

In a medium sauté pan over medium-low heat, heat the olive oil until hot but not smoking. Add the minced garlic and onion. Cook, stirring frequently, until soft and translucent. Add the sausage, and cook until lightly browned, about 3 minutes. Add the quinoa and stir constantly until lightly toasted, about 3 minutes. When the quinoa grains start to pop and look opaque, slowly stir in the evaporated skim milk and the chicken broth, stirring frequently for about 10 minutes, then add the bay leaf, fava beans, and morels, and continue cooking until slightly thickened, about another 10 minutes.

Turn off the heat, stir in the arugula, and cover. Let sit for 3 to 4 minutes. Check the risotto for salt and pepper, add the cheese, and serve.

Quinoa, an ancient Incan powerfood, may be an ingredient you're unfamiliar with, so I want to introduce you to it and its fabulous properties. Quinoa has been cultivated for more than five thousand years. Higher in protein than other grains, quinoa is also high in minerals such as iron and calcium, as well as B vitamins. Quinoa is an excellent source of energy fuel because of its high fiber content and quality complex carbohydrate composition, which is very low in simple sugars. Quinoa continues to be a sacred food for the Andean people because of its body-strengthening qualities. Eating whole grains—like quinoa—will curb your appetite for sugar since your body will be getting the carbohydrates it needs from a quality source.

Nutritional information per 1-person serving:

Serving	Calories	Total Fat	Carbs.	Fiber	Sugars	Antioxidant Protein	Rating
1 cup Quinoa Risotto Primavera topped with 1 tablespoon Manchego cheese	504	28.5g	26.3g	2g	2.9g	38.4g	1
1 cup Quinoa Risotto Primavera without cheese	384	18.5g	26.3g	2g	2.9g	30.5g	1
1 tablespoon Manchego cheese	120	10g	0	0	0	7.9g	1

Ensalada Girasol (Sunflower Salad)—Lunch

CHEF: ZARELA MARTÍNEZ   SERVES 4

● ●

LATIN POWER-FOODS

This beautiful and tasty salad combines the great flavors of broiled chicken, smoky chipotle, and sweet mango. It's also wonderfully adaptable—as I'm sure you'll discover (see note below). For a nonmeat version, use your favorite leafy greens and toss them with the vinaigrette-marinated mango and/or jícama. Garlic and chipotles (chiles) are the Latin power-foods in this recipe, and chicken is in the powerfood categories.

½ cup (or to taste) Pasta de Chipotle (see recipe below)

2 large whole boneless free-range chicken breasts with skin

2 to 4 tablespoons vegetable oil, or as needed

1 large mango (about 1 pound), peeled, seeded, and thinly sliced

2 cups Chipotle Vinaigrette (recipe follows)

First prepare the Pasta de Chipotle on page 142. Then preheat the oven broiler. Brush chipotle paste over both sides of the chicken breasts. Brush a little oil over the chipotle paste. Place on broiler pan and broil, skin side up, until skin starts to brown, about 4 minutes. Turn and broil for another 4 minutes. Turn off the broiler, reduce the oven heat to 400°F, and bake the chicken until cooked through, about 10 minutes longer. Let rest for 10 minutes for the juices to settle. Remove the skin, and slice on the bias.

Toss the sliced mango in the Chipotle Vinaigrette (see recipe below). Using tongs or a slotted spoon, lift out, letting the dressing drain back into the bowl. Arrange mango slices around 4 serving plates, sunflower-fashion. Toss the sliced chicken breasts in the remaining vinaigrette and pile in the center of the serving plates.

Note: Chef Zarela Martínez says that you can also include jícama. Just peel and cut it into a fine julienne or dice. Then, after slicing the chicken, toss jícama in the Chipotle Vinaigrette and lift it out with a slotted spoon, letting the dressing drain back into the bowl. Arrange jícama in center of serving plates. Continue with recipe, arranging sliced chicken on top of the jícama.

VINAGRETA DE CHIPOTLE (CHIPOTLE VINAIGRETTE)

This is a good dressing to experiment with. It would be great with a grilled duck salad or any green salad.

- ½ cup red wine vinegar
- 1 teaspoon garlic, minced
- 1 teaspoon Mexican oregano (available in Latin markets, large supermarkets, or online)

- 3 canned chipotle chiles en adobo (available in Latin markets, large supermarkets, or online), minced (or use fewer for milder flavor)
- salt and freshly ground black pepper
- 1 ½ cups olive oil

In a medium bowl, whisk together the vinegar, garlic, oregano, chipotle chiles, salt, and pepper. Add olive oil a little at a time, whisking well after each addition.

PASTA DE CHIPOTLE (CHIPOTLE PASTE)

- one 8-ounce can chipotle chiles en adobo (available in Latin markets, large supermarkets, or online)
- 4 to 5 garlic cloves, minced (about 2 tablespoons)

- 1 tablespoon dried Mexican oregano (available in Latin markets, large supermarkets, or online)
- 2 tablespoons olive oil

*E*mpty the 8-ounce can of chipotles and their sauce into a blender or food processor fitted with a steel blade. Process until puréed, about 1 minute. Add the garlic, oregano, and olive oil and process on pulse until combined but still slightly chunky. Use immediately, or store, tightly covered, in the refrigerator for up to 3 weeks.

Nutritional information per 1-person serving:

Serving	Calories	Total Fat	Carbs.	Fiber	Sugars	Protein	Antioxidant Rating
Ensalada Girasol with 6 ounces chicken with skin, with 1/2 cup mango, Chipotle Paste and Vinaigrette, including 1 tablespoon oil per serving	**520**	**28.6g**	**14g**	**2.1g**	**12.6g**	**44.6g**	**2**
2 tablespoons vinaigrette	240	26g	2g	0	0.5g	0	1
Ensalada Girasol without vinaigrette	**400**	**15.6g**	**13g**	**2.1g**	**12.3g**	**44.6g**	**1**
Ensalada Girasol with 1 cup greens instead of chicken, including paste and vinaigrette as listed above	225	13g	24g	5.4g	14.7g	4.7g	3

Note: Chipotle paste adds a negligible amount of calories, carbs, protein, fiber, and fat.

*C*hurrasco (Marinated Skirt Steak)—Dinner

CHEF: XIOMARA ARDOLINA   SERVES 4

● ●

LATIN POWER-FOODS

Easy to grill (stuff, roll, and braise!), skirt steak is found in many parts of the Americas. As in the case of most meat, it can be tough if it's not cooked properly. Marinating it as chef Xiomara Ardolina suggests will help yield tender and delicious results—without adding too much fat. Chef Ardolina recommends serving this dish with a leafy green salad and mashed potatoes with bleu cheese. This recipe has two of my Latin powerfoods, garlic and cilantro (or culantro). It also has onions, corn, and lean beef.

MARINADE

1 large onion, peeled and coarsely chopped

1 bunch of fresh cilantro, rinsed and coarsely chopped

1 cup vegetable oil

VEGETABLE MIXTURE

1 tablespoon vegetable oil

1 cup onions, diced

1 tablespoon garlic, minced

1 tablespoon fresh culantro (or cilantro)

½ cup porcini mushrooms, diced (if they're dry, they should be soaked and then chopped)

½ cup roasted corn kernels (you can grill them on the cob, or sauté them in a small pan until golden)

2 cups homemade or organic chicken stock

1 to 2 tablespoons *huitlacoche* (corn truffles, a Mexican delicacy, available canned in Latin markets, large supermarkets, or online)

½ tablespoon unsalted butter

salt and pepper to taste

four 8-ounce pieces of skirt steak

Combine the onion and cilantro in a food processor fitted with a metal blade. Slowly add the oil while blending. Combine the mixture in a bowl with the meat and cover. (You can also put both in a sealable bag.) Refrigerate for at least 10 minutes, or up to 1 day.

To prepare the vegetables, heat 1 tablespoon of vegetable oil in a large frying pan over medium heat. Add the onions, garlic, culantro, and porcini and sauté, stirring frequently, until the onions start to become transparent, about 3 minutes. Add the corn, then stir in the chicken stock and *huitlacoche* and let simmer until the mixture starts to reduce and reaches a medium consistency (not too thick, and not too thin), about 8 minutes. Stir in the butter. Season to taste.

To grill the meat, preheat a grill or large skillet over medium-high heat. Grill or fry the steaks for about 5 minutes per side, or to your desired degree of doneness. Remove from heat and let the meat rest for 5 to 10 minutes to let the juices settle. Cut each steak along the grain into 3 or 4 pieces. Set on a platter or individual serving plates with the sautéed vegetables. Serve immediately.

Nutritional information per 1-person serving:

	Serving	Calories	Total Fat	Carbs.	Fiber	Sugars	Protein	Antioxidant Rating
6 ounces skirt steak with ¼ cup marinade and ¼ cup vegetables		890	65g	10g	1g	2g	48g	1
Mashed Potatoes	1 cup	237	9g	35g	3g	3g	4g	2
Bleu Cheese	¼ cup	119	10g	1g	0	0	7g	1
Green Salad	2 cups	46	0	9g	4g	0	3g	2

Bistec Empanizado (Citrus and Spice—Marinated and Breaded Steak)—Dinner

CHEF: XIOMARA ARDOLINA   SERVES 6

● ●

LATIN POWER-FOODS

This is great with or without the addition of Japanese bread crumbs. Chef Xiomara Ardolina recommends serving her steak with black beans and white rice and a green leafy salad. This recipe has the Latin powerfood garlic, and lime and lean beef.

½ cup fresh lime juice

½ cup fresh orange juice

1 teaspoon fresh oregano

1 teaspoon ground cumin

1 teaspoon garlic, chopped

salt and pepper to taste

6 pieces top sirloin, pounded about ¼ inch thick

2 eggs, beaten

3 cups panko (Japanese bread crumbs)

1 tablespoon canola or olive oil (more as needed)

6 lime wedges (one for each steak)

½ cup fresh parsley leaves, chopped

In a large ceramic or Pyrex dish, combine the citrus juices, oregano, cumin, and garlic. Add salt and pepper and stir well. Add the steaks, and mix so that the meat is well coated with the citrus sauce, cover, and refrigerate for at least 10 minutes, and up to a few hours.

To prepare the meat for cooking, lift out of the marinade with tongs and set onto a platter. Pour the eggs into a recessed plate. Do the same with the bread crumbs. Take one piece of the steak and coat it in egg first. Let drain, and dip it into the bread crumbs, making sure that the meat is well covered on both sides. Place on a plate. Repeat with the remaining pieces of steak.

Heat the oil in a medium skillet over medium-high heat. Cook the meat, in batches as needed, until nice and brown and at your desired degree of doneness. Garnish with lime and parsley, and serve.

Nutritional information per 1-person serving:

	Serving	Calories	Total Fat	Carbs.	Fiber	Sugars	Protein	Antioxidant Rating
6 ounces marinated and breaded steak		607	17g	46g	2.6g	3.5g	44.3g	1
Black beans and rice	1 cup	340	10g	33g	16g	2g	7g	2
Green salad	2 cups	46	0	9g	4g	0	3g	2

Grilled Vegetables with Cilantro Pesto—Snack

CHEF: SUE TORRES

SERVES 4 TO 6

● ●

LATIN POWER-FOODS

This recipe is really three in one: You've got the fabulous Cilantro Pesto (this stuff is marvelous on top of fresh tomatoes, grilled chicken—you name it!), Pico de Gallo—another easily adaptable salsa—and, of course, the grilled veggies. As chef Sue Torres says, this is really a left-over snack! In other words, this could be served as a lunch one day, and then a snack the next. This snack combines three Latin power-foods: chiles, cilantro, and garlic. It also has pine nuts, onion, tomato, and lime.

CILANTRO PESTO

1 cup packed fresh cilantro leaves and stems, chopped

1 clove garlic, thinly sliced

1 cup oil

1/8 cup toasted pine nuts

2 teaspoons salt or to taste

PICO DE GALLO

2 cups tomatoes, seeded, cut into 1/4-inch dice

1 cup white (or Spanish) onion, cut into 1/4-inch dice

2 or 3 serrano chiles, stemmed and diced (seeds and all)

1/3 cup fresh lime juice

2 tablespoons fresh cilantro, chopped

1 teaspoon salt or to taste

GRILLED VEGETABLES

1 teaspoon salt

1 teaspoon black pepper

1 serrano cut into ⅛-inch-thick circles, seeds and all

2 green zucchinis, cut lengthwise into ¼-inch-thick slices (so that you have nice long strips that won't fall through the grill)

2 yellow zucchini, cut lengthwise into ¼-inch-thick slices

2 chayote (Mexican squash), peeled, sliced into ¼-inch-thick slices, and seeded (or you can let the pit fall out when it's grilling)

1 teaspoon garlic, minced

4 to 6 cilantro sprigs, for garnish

*T*o make the pesto, combine the cilantro, garlic, and ⅓ cup of the oil in a blender. Pulse several times until it starts to purée. Add the pine nuts, and slowly pour in ¼ cup more of the oil. Add salt. Set aside, or cover and store in an airtight container in the refrigerator for up to 3 days.

To make the Pico de Gallo, combine all of the ingredients in a medium-size bowl. Cover with plastic wrap and let sit at room temperature for an hour. Taste and adjust seasoning if necessary. Serve or store in an airtight container in the refrigerator for up to 3 days.

To grill the vegetables, preheat grill to medium-high heat. In a medium-size bowl, combine the remaining oil and the salt and pepper with the serrano slices and stir well. Lay your veggies on a sheet pan, and using a pastry brush coat each side with the garlic and the chile-oil mixture. Flip and brush the other side. Grill until marked on both sides (and until the veggies become limp), about 2 to 4 minutes per side.

Slice the grilled veggies horizontally into ⅛-inch-wide strips. Divide into serving dishes. Top each serving with a spoonful of Pico de Gallo, and small dollops (about 2 tablespoons per person) of Cilantro Pesto. Top with a sprig of cilantro, and serve. (Vegetables can be warm, or at room temperature, or chilled.)

	Serving	Calories	Total Fat	Carbs.	Fiber	Sugars	Protein	Antioxidant Rating
Grilled Vegetables with 2 tablespoons Cilantro Pesto and 1 tablespoon Pico de Gallo		375	35g	14g	6g	4g	9g	2
Grilled Vegetables	1 cup	70	7g	8g	3g	0	2g	2
Cilantro Pesto 2 tablespoons		300	28g	6g	2g	4g	7g	2

Note: *Pico de Gallo adds a negligible amount of calories, carbs, protein, fiber, and fat.*

Crisp Toasts with Chimichurri—Snack

CHEF: ARLEN GARGAGLIANO   MAKES ABOUT 1¼ CUPS CHIMICHURRI

● ●

LATIN POWER-FOODS

Not unlike a pesto, this sauce, which comes from Argentina, is an ever-present condiment in parilladas *(barbecued meat restaurants). Arlen says she continues to find ways to use her chimichurri! Wonderful as a marinade, or dipping sauce, or served atop a grilled piece of chicken or fish, it's also nice spread on crisp toasts (as described here), fresh tomatoes (and mozzarella!), grilled potatoes—and so much more! You can vary the herb balance depending on what you like and what you have available. This snack has the Latin powerfood garlic.*

1 long French-style baguette, preferably whole wheat, sliced into ¼-inch-thick rounds, and then halved into half-moon-shaped pieces

3 cloves garlic (or to taste), chopped

leaves from 1 sprig of oregano

2 bay leaves

2 teaspoons sweet paprika

leaves from 6 sprigs of thyme

15 basil leaves

1 bunch fresh parsley, coarsely chopped, plus additional chopped parsley for garnish

½ teaspoon cumin seeds

kosher salt and freshly ground pepper to taste

½ cup white balsamic vinegar

¾ cup olive oil

Preheat the oven to 350°F. Spread the bread rounds on a baking sheet. Toast for about 10 minutes on each side, or until lightly browned. Let cool and store in an airtight container until you're ready to use them.

Combine all the remaining ingredients, except for the parsley garnish, in a food processor or a blender and process till smooth. Use the chimichurri immediately, or cover and refrigerate for up to 1 week. Return to room temperature and mix well prior to serving. To prepare the tostadas, set the bread rounds on a platter and spread the chimichurri (usually, since it's liquidy, Arlen uses a small espresso-size spoon) on top. Sprinkle with chopped parsley and serve immediately.

Nutritional information per 1-person serving:

	Serving	Calories	Total Fat	Carbs.	Fiber	Sugars	Protein	Antioxidant Rating
½ cup Chimichurri with 1 cup Crisp Toasts		250	9.5g	38g	2g	3g	6.5g	2
Chimichurri	½ cup	100	8g	8g	1g	2g	0.5g	2
Crisp Toasts	1 cup	150	1.5g	30g	1g	1g	6g	1

Pepitas (Toasted Pumpkin Seeds)—Snack

CHEF: ARLEN GARGAGLIANO   MAKES 1 CUP (ABOUT FOUR SERVINGS)

● ●

LATIN POWER-FOODS

Perfect any time of year, these crunchy treats can be adjusted depending on how much you like to spice it up! Easy to store, these are great taken along to work (or school!) in a sealed container—or served in a pretty ceramic dish. Chipotle and garlic are the Latin powerfoods in this dish.

1 cup raw pumpkin seeds

3 cloves garlic or to taste, crushed

1 chipotle en adobo, finely diced (you can also purée the can of chipotles, and use about ½ teaspoon of the purée or according to taste)

¼ teaspoon kosher salt or to taste

1 teaspoon turbinado sugar

1 lime wedge

*H*eat a medium-size heavy frying pan, and pour in the pumpkin seeds. Let toast for about 5 minutes, stirring constantly. Stir in the garlic and cook for another 2 minutes. Add the chipotle, salt, and sugar and mix well so that all the seeds are coated. Remove from heat and pour into a bowl. Serve immediately, or let cool and store in an airtight container for up to 1 week. Before serving, squeeze the wedge of lime on top.

Nutritional information per 1-person serving:

	Serving	Calories	Total Fat	Carbs.	Fiber	Sugars	Protein	Antioxidant Rating
Pepitas	¼ cup	294	23.1g	8g	2.3g	2g	18.9g	1

TRACK THREE RECAP

Congratulations! You've successfully reached the final stage of the Hot Latin Diet, which is all about maintaining a healthy lifestyle. I hope you are satisfied with your progress, and that you have reached your ideal weight by now. But more important, I hope you have managed to incorporate the Hot Latin lifestyle philosophy and make it your own. Hopefully you have found new ways to bring the seven Latin powerfoods into your daily diet, and a whole new world of culinary possibilities has opened up to you.

It is absolutely normal to fall off the wagon sometimes. During the holidays, a vacation, or a particularly crazy week at work, we've all had to forget our healthy eating objectives just in order to get by. And if this happens to you, know that you are not alone, and as I've said before, it's definitely not something worth punishing yourself for. If a few weeks have gone by, and you feel that you've started to gain weight, just put an end to it right away, and go back to Track One for two weeks, and that will be enough to get you back on track and feeling good about yourself.

GUIDELINES FOR MAINTAINING A HEALTHY LIFESTYLE

☑ *Guidelines for the Spirit*

☑ *Guidelines for Nutrition*

☑ *Guidelines for Exercise*

A_s *I said from day one, changing your lifestyle is not* easy. It's tough because so many of us face everyday situations that make it really difficult to stay the course. (And let's not mention those eight factors that contribute to weight gain!) Sometimes no matter how much we plan, unexpected bumps in the road cause us to deviate. When it comes to dieting, these bumps can also steer us back to our old, unhealthy ways.

I can't help but think of something that I often hear from my pregnant patients, and it relates here as far as absolutes go. Many times, my new mothers will request, "Dr. Manny, please, no matter what I say, I don't want any painkillers when I give birth to my baby; I want to be totally drug-free." Though this is certainly commendable, it's not always realistic—but it's hard to say that to ambitious moms (and dads!) when they're trying to do the right thing. And in cases where my patients have had to go back on their original statements—because of things like back labor and other situations beyond their control—they often feel defeated, though I try to tell them that they shouldn't.

The same is true with a diet. If you set yourself up with absolutes, you're bound to suffer! If you've followed my advice up to now, you've cleaned your fridge, you've gotten rid of those pantry temptations and replaced them with healthful ingredients, and you're now following the three tracks of this diet and reaping the benefits of eating the seven Latin powerfoods. Basically, you're working your way to a long-lasting healthy lifestyle. So why would you set yourself up with absolutes? My advice is to not do this. Perfection is a tough ideal in the world of dieting; trying your best is the path to take.

Below I've listed the most important guidelines to follow in keeping up with your new lifestyle. To maintain a healthy balance, it is crucial to pay attention to the needs of your spirit, mind, and body.

Guidelines for the Spirit

KEEP THAT MOTIVATION HIGH

As we learned in the beginning of this diet, having a good attitude and approach is just as crucial to the success of a diet as is eating healthy and getting enough exercise. Here are some suggestions to keep that motivation train running on the right track.

✔ THE BIG C: CONFIDENCE

Though it comes from within, it shows on the outside. With achievements—goals attained, even if they're small—you should feel more confidence (poise and assurance), and that's a good thing, because you'll feel better and you'll notice that people react positively to you. Hold that beautiful head high, my friend.

✔ CELEBRATE YOUR ACHIEVEMENTS

Even the smallest of achievements—the loss of a couple of pounds, the implementation of a new exercise routine, that glow of healthiness—deserves recognition. Get yourself a manicure, or how about a massage? Go buy that book you've been dying to get your hands on. Do something to commemorate your efforts—but make sure it's not chocolate cake!

✔ THAT BEAUTIFUL DRESS

Remember that dress you set aside for when you could fit into it the way you want to? You know—the way that shows off your curves at just the right angles? Take that baby out, and even though you may not be there yet, give yourself a smile—and a promise—that you're getting there . . . and that soon you'll be wearing it and seeing how gorgeous it looks on *you*, instead of on that hanger!

LEARN TO DEAL WITH STRESS

If you're like me—and many of my patients—it may be stress that often leads you to eat poorly. Therefore, because stress is often a catalyst in our eating habits, part of changing your attitude is also changing the cycle of how you might react to certain stress-producing situations. Your awareness of this is especially important as you start your new diet. But before we get into this, I need to elaborate a bit on the stress thing.

Most of us equate stress with that neck-knotting, fingernail-biting, over-the-top pressure and tension. After a disturbing—or tragic—event in our lives, our stress is what helps or hinders our adjustment to new circumstances. As negative stress progresses, it can translate into a myriad of bad feelings—like anger, rejection, distrust, and depression. If these escalate further, your bad stress can lead to a whole host of health problems, ranging from headaches to heart disease. Yet another little-known consequence of negative stress is obesity; in some cases, chronic stress can lead to the increase in a hormone called cortisol, which contributes to the formation of fat.

On the other hand, there's positive stress. This kind of stress can really help you, especially as you're embarking on changes as big as diet and lifestyle. Positive stress can bring passion, motivation, anticipation, and excitement to life—and these are the qualities that many of us thrive with. So the key here is to find your "best" stress level, and work with it. Again, this isn't easy—especially when we really have a tough time with change.

Identifying unrelieved stress and knowing how it affects you is simply not enough for eliminating its consequences. Luckily there are many different ways of managing it. The key is twofold: changing the source of stress (which may or may not always be possible), and, more important, changing your reaction to it.

For example, so many of us who would like to lose weight or change our bodies are knee-jerk eaters: as soon as we're stressed, tired, unhappy, or just whiney, we reach for those chocolate chips.

So I'm going to give you some phrases to help change the way you think—to deflate that bad-stress anxiety balloon and jump-start your good-stress, positive thinking.

▶ *Instead of:* Why did this have to happen?

☺ **Try: What should I learn from this?**

▶ *Instead of:* I can't deal with this.

☺ **Try: What steps should I take to relieve this stress?**

▶ *Instead of:* This is a difficult problem.

☺ **Try: How can I best meet this challenge?**

▶ *Instead of:* I can't possibly solve this.

☺ **Try: Who could help me find a solution?**

It's hard not to fall back into repeated patterns of thought and expression; it definitely requires effort. Here, the idea of making a positive out of a negative is one that has helped me—and my patients—achieve goals.

RESERVE SOME TIME FOR RELAXING

It is very important to take time each day for relaxation and recuperation. I recommend even just taking five minutes before sitting up and getting out of bed in the morning and before going to sleep at night: Close your eyes and take twenty deep, full, slow breaths through your mouth. Imagine that with each breath out you're clearing your mind and releasing tension from your body, and that you are focused on how you feel in the present moment, and with each breath in imagine yourself energized and present. This is a great way to connect with yourself and to feel more clear and grounded throughout your day. You can do this breathing technique as often as you wish, especially any time you are feeling stressed or upset. Taking yoga classes is a fabulous way to become fit as well as to reduce stress because of its meditative quality. You can also take time to stretch each day. A simple way to approach stretching is to just move your body in every possible way you can without straining. For instance, move your wrist in every possible way it can move, and do the same with your ankle, and so on, and apply this to every joint and body part, while also gently stretching with each movement in this range of motion.

SET UP A REGULAR ROUTINE FOR SLEEP

I always suggest trying to keep a regular routine going. In my case, I know I've got to get up at five every day, so I try to hit the hay no later than eleven p.m. Studies have proven, in fact, that you are more likely to get a good night's rest when your body is accustomed to a routine (especially one in which you're sleeping a decent number of hours—and by that I mean at least six). I also suggest using the bed for sleeping—and not for watching TV or working on your laptop. Also, don't go to bed hungry, and don't exercise three hours before bedtime (when your body could still be stimulated). If you're fading during the day, give yourself time for a fifteen-minute power nap to help you catch up a bit. (And naps can even be longer on weekends!)

LEARN TO FORGIVE YOURSELF

If you do gain a couple of pounds, don't beat yourself up about it! It happens from time to time—and then you make up for it. Again, the trick—as we've discussed and our chefs have concurred—is that you can't deny yourself, but you can control yourself. I'm a firm believer in the three-bite rule. Do you know this one? This is when you can take three bites of anything! Okay, I mean you still have to keep your wits about you—but you can try that luscious dessert without eating the whole thing, right?

And when your scale moves upward, or those pants start to feel a bit tighter around the hips and waist, you know exactly what to do: take control. You've done it before, and you'll do it again. Get right back on this Hot Latin Diet—start with Track One, and you'll be back on track to your gorgeous figure in no time.

Top Ways to Maintain Your Desired Weight!

- ✔ Keep tempting foods out of your cupboards (remember: out of sight, out of mind)!

- ✔ Don't let yourself feel deprived! Eat a variety of foods to get all the nutrients you need. Include choices from whole grains, fruits, vegetables, and lean protein sources. (Check out our recipes and nutritional charts, as well as snacking tips!)

- ✔ Don't skip meals! Not only can it slow down your metabolism, it can also lead you to overeat during the latter part of the day.

- ✔ Eat only when you're hungry and do something else when you're not.

✔ Try to keep food out of the emotional equation; learn to deal with problems without relying on food.

✔ Keep moving! Physical activity—primarily because it boosts your metabolism—is one of the most important aspects of keeping weight off. Make setting aside time—at least twenty minutes for physical activity every day—part of your natural schedule. Write it down so you can keep a record of what you're doing (and celebrate your accomplishments)!

✔ Keep your eye on the scale. If the number is going up, take that as a warning, and start to make some adjustments.

✔ Create a food journal. Make sure you're writing everything down. This will help increase your awareness of exactly what you're eating and drinking, as well as what changes you may need to make as time goes on.

Top Reasons Why Diets Don't Work

1. The search for a quick fix instead of long-term changes
2. Eating mindlessly
3. I'm stressed: Let's eat
4. Heading for fries instead of an apple . . .
5. Caving in to others' needs instead of your own
6. The ol' "I'll start my diet tomorrow"
7. Hitting the bottle
8. Taking a drastic all-or-nothing approach
9. Thinking, "I can't"

Guidelines for Nutrition

CHOOSE QUALITY OVER QUANTITY

To succeed with the Hot Latin Diet, you have to choose the best quality ingredients. Many of our chefs say their choices for eating are market-driven; they go to the store and see what's seasonal and available, and take it from there. This, along with the other tips I've given you throughout the book, is smart living. The Hot Latin Diet promotes mouthwatering recipes and combinations of flavors by using fresh seasonal ingredients, natural condiments, herbs, and spices. I prefer that you choose organic food, or the best quality available to you. I advocate the inclusion of any and all of our seven Latin powerfood categories, and especially our seven Latin powerfoods: garbanzos, tomatillos, avocados, chiles, cinnamon, garlic, and cilantro—which will help your body stay working at optimal levels, keep your skin healthy, your eyes bright, and you looking hot!

Remember, this diet does not exclude any food group; I believe all foods are important and that variety plays a fundamental role in healthy eating. Someone once gave me excellent advice that I'd like to pass along to you: When grocery shopping, fill your cart with items from the periphery of the store, where you'll find fish, fruit, veggies, and fresh whole-grain breads. Look for all-natural and organic items and stay far away from processed foods.

PAY ATTENTION TO PORTION SIZES

The exact size of portions to eat daily will vary depending on how many calories you choose to consume, but again I suggest not dropping below 1,800 calories a day. Whether you choose 2,500, 2,000, or 1,800 calories, I recommend maintaining equal ratios in terms of proteins, fats, and carbohydrates; in other words, do not favor one category of food over others. The best bet is to eat a balanced diet daily, according to the chart below. If you want to eat lighter, increase the amount of raw salads, green vegetables, fruits, and water you drink, while reducing other foods across the board. The calorie content for each food is available in the seven powerfoods charts on pages 15–18. You can experiment with the serving amounts to figure out what exact combination works best for you each day, and trust your instincts about what your body tells you it needs. This will be easier to do over time as you follow my guidelines. You will be able to listen to your body's signals once you have a structure in place. Remember to eat something every three to four hours, and spread out your servings and types of foods throughout the day. Vegetarians can increase portions of beans, tubers, and grains by one to two servings per day in place of animal proteins. The calorie content per serving is approximate, since each food within each category varies in caloric content. Do not worry about this. What I am envisioning for you is, again, a lifestyle, not a number-crunching preoccupation. The body does not operate simply in terms of calories, but also in terms of calorie quality—so if you eat wholesome natural foods you will do just fine.

Visualizing Portion Sizes

▶ One serving of vegetables: the size of your fist

▶ One serving of rice or pasta: the size of one scoop of ice cream

▶ One serving of meat, fish, or poultry: the size of your palm (without your fingers!) or a deck of cards

▶ One serving of snacks (such as nuts): the size of a cupped handful

▶ Apple: the size of a baseball

FOOD PORTION SIZE CHART

Food Group	Serving Size	Calories/Day 1,800	2,000	2,500
Fruit	1 whole medium-size fruit, or 1 cup sliced fruit, or 1 cup fresh fruit juice	1	2	2–3
Vegetables and Chiles	1 cup raw salad or 1 cup cooked veg. or 1 cup fresh veg.	4	5	6
Beans	1 cup cooked beans	1	2	3
Grains and Tubers	2 slices sprouted grain bread or 1 cup cooked grain or tuber	1	2	3
Oils	1 tablespoon high-quality organic olive or vegetable oil	2	2	2
Raw Nuts	1/3 cup raw nuts	1	2	2
Animal Meats	6 ounces lean meat, poultry, or seafood	1	1–1.5	1–1.5
Eggs	2 medium organic eggs	No more than 2 to 3 servings per week for all calorie intakes		
Dairy	1 cup organic low-fat milk or yogurt, or 4 ounces cheese	No more than 1 to 2 servings per week for all calorie intakes		
Spices and Herbs	Enjoy to taste as long as all-natural, low-salt, and preservative- and sugar-free			

OTHER TIPS FOR PORTION CONTROL

Portion is also controlled by the way in which meals are delivered to you. Check out the size of your plates. If they're ten-inchers, you're probably eating more than you should, simply because of the plate size. So take it down; try eating off of eight- or even six-inch plates. The same is true with your eating tools; if you're using larger utensils (come on—we've all scooped up mashed potatoes, and then eaten them, with a serving spoon), you should move to the smaller spoons and salad forks. Of course, you could go with chopsticks!

SLOW IT DOWN

Another factor in portion control is speed. Have you ever timed yourself to see how much time you take to eat a meal? So many of us are on the superfast line for everything—including scarfing down meals. This is *not* a good thing; as I've mentioned before, timing is everything. What's happening when you're inhaling your food is that your stomach doesn't even have time to tell you you're full—because you're still too busy shoveling it in and you're not getting the message in time. The bottom line is you've got to slow it down! Believe it or not, it takes about twenty minutes for your stomach to send your brain the "full" signal. This means that if you're not taking it slower, you're definitely overeating. And there are other consequences to the food-gulping thing: you can throw your body off the proper digestive track—and actually give yourself gas, among other stomach woes—if you don't let the body begin its natural process of producing digestive enzymes and beginning its natural course of processing your food.

KNOW WHEN TO EAT

I once told a patient, "If you really want to lose weight, stop eating after six!" You know what? It worked! But in order to do this, you may have to shift your whole day's meals. Here's a possible timing scenario: If you eat your breakfast at about eight, you should have a snack around ten thirty, then lunch at noon, a snack at about three, and dinner at around six.

If this is all too early for you, try shifting it up a bit—but you don't want to eat too late at night; after eight your body goes into a different rhythm, and your metabolism starts to slow down. I suggest eating your last meal of the day a solid two to three hours prior to sleeping.

If you've traveled to Latin America, you may have noticed one big difference in terms of the timing of the big meal of the day: we Latinos typically eat our biggest meal during the day (as opposed to in the evening). There's a lot of emphasis on eating bigger meals—breakfast and lunch—earlier in the day. But now you're going to say, "I've been to Argentina and seen how they eat dinner at ten at night!" Yes—but if they do, they're eating meals that are high in protein and low in carbs. My advice to you is to try to eat dinner before seven or seven thirty (or approximately three hours before you go to bed). This can be tough to do, especially if you're like many of us who suffer from late-night food cravings. But I urge you, when the mood hits and you want a sweet snack, reach for something other than that ice cream. Keeping fresh fruit on hand is very helpful during these times.

Also, please don't skip your morning meal! I don't think a Latino household would let its occupants leave without breakfast. Seriously, breakfast is so important for us because it jump-starts our metabolism and gets us ready for all of the work—both physical and mental—we have to tackle. In fact, studies show that people who eat breakfast—versus those who skip breakfast—actually burn more calories. Also, eating a good breakfast will keep you from getting too hungry, which, in turn, leads to overeating. Again, by putting fuel in your tank, you're keeping your appetite on an even keel, which will help you control impulsive eating when your emotions start to get the best of you. It's actually been proven that many of us (especially women) eat less compulsively if we've had breakfast. But in case you needed even more support for my advice, consider this: eating breakfast will help your mental performance. A study published in the November 2001 issue of the *American Journal of Clinical Nutrition* showed that eating breakfast improved participants' performance on memory tests.

SPREAD OUT YOUR MEALS, AND DON'T FORGET TO SNACK!

How often you eat is as big a concern as how much—and your metabolism is an important body process to keep first and foremost in your mind. There are several factors that influence your ability to convert the fuel in your food into the energy needed to power everything you do, ranging from exercise (or lack thereof) to when and how much you eat. For example, if you think you're doing yourself a favor by skipping breakfast, think again; not eating breakfast will keep your metabolism low. In fact, this first meal of the day not only gets you going, it can also help to lessen your appetite throughout the day. I recommend eating one of the breakfast plans in this diet or a combination of organic oatmeal plus fruit—like mangoes, papayas, blueberries, raspberries, nectarines, or melon. Think seasonally—and organically—whenever possible.

And once breakfast is over, that doesn't mean starving yourself until dinner; snacking will actually prevent you from getting that I-have-to-eat-something-right-now feeling. This is important, because I'm sure you know that the hungrier you are, the less control you have over what and how much you eat. Also, keeping your metabolism high involves snacking; the important thing, of course, is that you pick healthy snacks. Choose complex carbohydrates (like fresh fruits, vegetables, and grains) to fuel your metabolism. I recommend having two to three snacks per day, limiting them to about 250 calories apiece (but make sure they're healthy calories!).

If you're on the road and looking for a quick snack fix, don't succumb, my friend, to those sugary candy bars posing as energy bars that are now on counters everywhere. Check the ingredients; make sure they're as natural as possible. If there are a lot of words you don't recognize, they may be chemicals. Go with ones that don't have too many ingredients—the ones with simple things that are understandable.

There are healthy choices for bars that you can grab and go with. For example, I really like the spirulina bars (spirulina is a vitamin-, mineral-, and nutrient-packed blue-green freshwater algae, which is a great source of protein, antioxidants, and essential fatty acids) available in health-food stores. Or raw fruit bars, or dried fruit and nut bars, many of which are not only packed with vitamins, but also taste good. These may not be as readily available where you are, so perhaps you will have to plan ahead; order them online, or go to a health-food store, one of the big health-food chains, or one of the vitamin stores—I promise it will be worth it!

ENJOY ALCOHOL IN MODERATION

If you've traveled to Latin America, you know that we enjoy cocktails—along with snacking and chatting. You couldn't possibly leave Peru without trying their luscious Pisco Sours—their national drink—with, of course, a side dish of *anticuchos*, marinated and roasted skewered beef; or Brazil without enjoying a fresh lime-packed *caipirinha* along-side a small selection of *pão de queijo*, small fresh-baked soft rolls of manioc (yuca) flour and light cheese.

The philosophy behind cocktails and snacks in Latin America is one I adhere to and espouse whether we're talking cocktails or food: it's all about balance. Please know that when I mention alcohol, I'm talking about it in moderation; I certainly do not recommend more than two hard liquor beverages a week, but a glass of red wine at dinner can aid digestion, help lower bad cholesterol, and provide you with antioxi-dants along with your meal. If you do not already drink wine with your meals, I am not prompting you to start, but for those of you who enjoy a glass of red wine, or occasional white wine, keep moderation in mind.

If you do drink alcohol, just know that alcohol is the first source of fuel that the body will burn before turning to proteins, fats, and carbo-hydrates from foods. Also, alcohol can be hard on the liver to metabo-lize. And, despite a few health benefits from red wine, the carbohydrates in alcohol are all simple sugar carbs—not the healthiest kind. Snacking while sipping cocktails is key; you shouldn't drink alcohol on an empty stomach. In fact, several biochemical studies confirm that eating should accompany drinking (alcohol); in addition to slowing down the absorption process, which keeps blood-alcohol levels lower, moderate consumption during or around mealtime may have even favorable effects on digestion. Most countries in Latin America boast their own cocktail and—of course—accompanying snack.

Basically my rule for mixing cocktails is the same as for preparing food: use fresh and excellent-quality ingredients. There's a whole movement now toward the healthy cocktail. Many hip hangouts now boast blends of not only herbal-infused high-quality alcohols, but also the infusion of everything from the famous antioxidant Brazilian berry açaí, to other curative passion fruit and guava mixtures. Not too long ago, the U.S. Department of Agriculture reported that by combining strawberries and blackberries with alcohol, the antioxidant qualities of the fruits are actually enhanced.

Of course, I have to tell you that alcohol combined with anything is still alcohol, and you need to be aware of its consequences (did I say moderation?). However, if you're going to do some imbibing, I say do it Latin style—and pack your cocktails with top-shelf healthy fruits and flavors. Again, the quality of all components of the cocktail are always important to consider. For example, in the Caribbean, we've got a plethora of cocktails that include not only fresh fruit but also herbs—and even spices. Just look at *mojitos* (yes, a rum drink from my native Cuba!) made with fresh lime juice and mint leaves (and not too much sugar, *por favor*). This cocktail is not only wonderfully refreshing, it's also packed with antioxidants. Or how about a ginger-lemonade cocktail, made with the oh-so-curative and tasty fresh ginger, combined with light flavors of freshly squeezed lemon? All of the drinks I've mentioned here have something in common: they're made with alcohol alongside fresh ingredients—and never sugary (and often artificial) prepackaged mixes.

Of course, no discussion of alcohol could possibly be complete without touching on one of my favorites: wine. These days it's so easy to find a delicious Argentine Malbec, or a Chilean Cabernet Sauvignon—and so many more. I'm delighted to know that this luscious liquid is not only tasty and hugely complementary when matched appropriately to all kinds of dishes, but that it's also a healthy companion to dinners.

Not too long ago, I reported findings based on a Danish study. This new study, based on the self-reported drinking habits of some fifty-seven thousand middle-aged Danes, shows that the more women drink—and the more often men drink—the healthier their hearts. The study was conducted by the Center for Alcohol Research at Denmark's National Institute for Public Health.

Now I'm not saying that nondrinkers should change their ways—nor am I advocating that drinkers increase the amount they're consuming—but I do want to make you aware of a few things. Just to reiterate, excessive drinking and binge drinking can contribute to raising blood pressure, cause heart failure, and lead to a stroke. Furthermore, it can contribute to cancer and other diseases, and even obesity.

However, as we Latinos have known for years, drinking in moderation has benefits! In fact, other doctors have spoken up about this: Dr. Dawn Kershner, a cardiologist with Mid-Atlantic Cardiovascular Associates at Union Memorial Hospital in Baltimore, said she advises her patients to drink in moderation and to limit their drinking to no more than two drinks per day. She said a regular glass of wine can act as a blood thinner and raise good cholesterol. Whether we're talking food or cocktails, we need to be responsible. Balance, as always, is key.

Here is a chart that shows you how many calories are present in several drinks, and a reasonable weekly consumption amount—a total of five glasses of wine a week, or maybe two beers, or two mixed or hard liquor servings a week maximum.

ALCOHOL CALORIES

Type of Alcohol	Calorie Content	Carbohydrate Content	Maximum Consumption per week
red wine	164 per 6-oz. glass	6.5g	5 glasses
rosé wine	122 per 6-oz. glass	3.2g	3 glasses
white wine	160 per 6-oz. glass	9g	4 glasses
champagne	117 per 6-oz. glass	1.8g	4 glasses
port	188 per 4-oz. glass	14.4g	1 glass
light beer	145 per 12-oz. bottle	10.6g	2 beers
dark beer	126 per 12-oz. bottle	10g	2 beers
"diet" beer	96 per 12-oz. bottle	3.2g	2 beers
whiskey	128 per 2-oz. glass	0g	2 servings
vodka	128 per 2-oz. glass	0g	2 servings
gin	128 per 2-oz. glass	0g	2 servings
rum	128 per 2-oz. glass	0g	2 servings
tequila	128 per 2-oz. glass	0g	2 servings
sweet liqueurs	182 per 2-oz. glass	30g	1 serving
classic martini	139 per 4-oz. cocktail glass	0g	1 serving
gin and tonic	135 per 2-oz. gin plus tonic	1g	1 serving
rum and coke	208 per 2-oz. rum plus 6-oz. Coke	20g	1 serving
margarita	157 per 4-oz. cocktail glass	7g	1 serving
piña colada	328 per 6-oz. glass	42g	1 serving
vodka and fruit juice	214 per 2-oz. vodka and 6-oz. juice	19g	1 serving

Remember, if you are having a drink, to factor alcohol calories into your daily caloric intake, and if you know you are going to a cocktail party, then you can save some calories the day before to compensate.

Do not attempt to drink on an empty stomach, as this will simply make you hungrier later and then all your willpower and dedication will go out the window.

The day following an event where you might have a couple of drinks, aim to eat lots of fresh green salads and vegetables, and drink plenty of filtered or spring water to cleanse your body.

STICK TO YOUR DIET

One thing that's tough for all of us is sticking to a diet when we're, well, living real life! Actually this—the fact that many diets don't consider your real life—is my major complaint with many of 'em. But the Hot Latin Diet is different in that it's flexible and easy to follow. So before you cancel your night out with the girls and boys, or dinner with the boss and company, or your neighbor's party, check out these tips.

✔ DON'T STARVE YOURSELF!

It's four o'clock. You've got a dinner engagement at seven, and you are soooooo hungry. What can you do? Answer: Have a snack! Of course, you should have been eating all day (our suggested meals and snacks) as well as complementing your food with plenty of glasses of refreshing water. In fact, if you follow the Hot Latin Diet, you won't have that crazy craving-food-right-now feeling because you'll be keeping yourself sated with healthy calories.

✔ WHEN YOU'RE OUT, MAKE SURE YOU GET THOSE DRESSINGS AND SAUCES ON THE SIDE.

You know the drill: those non-health-conscious restaurants may bathe your salads—and meats—with sugar-packed dressings and sauces.

Stay away from them! Stick to the real food as much as possible. Yes, lemon or lime may not be as exciting as dressing, but combining it with just a bit of oil does bring out the best in fresh greens. Also, have your veggies raw or steamed (or lightly sautéed), and your lean meats or fish poached, broiled, baked, grilled, or roasted. As far as sauces go, I'd steer clear unless you know more about them (as in what ingredients they're made of). You've read this far in the book, so you know what to do! Use the judgment we've been working on.

✔ STEER AWAY FROM THOSE FATTY FOODS!

This is a tough one. You're at a cocktail party and the waiter is enticing you with the cheesy puffs (as if their beautiful aroma weren't enough). Unless you know you can handle having just a couple, I say don't do it. Go for the crudités; you'll feel much better eating the veggies . . . and your slimming body will thank you.

✔ IF IT'S YOUR BEST FRIEND'S BIRTHDAY,

FOR GOODNESS' SAKE, TAKE A SMALL PIECE OF CAKE!

If you just say no, no, *no* to every treat that passes you by, you're going to end up going crazy and your friends and family are going to go crazy. So, think moderation—as always—and balance. Again, use your best and newfound diet judgment, and don't beat yourself up!

DURING THE HOLIDAYS

For many of us, getting through the holidays is like walking through a food minefield. We Latinos take our holiday festivities very seriously—and we start in early December, and finish on January 6!— so I totally empathize with you as far as how tough it is to resist the temptations during this season. One of the keys to keeping that gorgeous figure of yours is to continue using your food as your ally—not your enemy. With the right foods, you should be okay. Let me give you some other tips to arm yourself with; and though my focus here is on the holiday season, you could use many of these ideas any time! Here are a few ideas for you.

HOLIDAY STRESS TIP

You and I both know that eating can be a response to emotions, and that stress often contributes to weight gain. The trick here is to not let it all get to you! Try to get your sleep (very important as far as keeping your positive outlook and staying healthy), not to overdo it in the area of alcohol (and food, of course!), "big picture" it all, and organize yourself so that you're prepared for this crazy time of year. Prioritize so that you're doing what's most important first, and you don't get caught up in that everyday minutiae. Don't go back to your old habits and cave in to the emotional eating that sometimes takes us over. Keep plenty of healthy foods on hand so that when your knee-jerk reaction is to reach for food, you come up with something good for you!

HOLIDAY PARTY TIP

I'm sure you've done the ol' supermarket run on an empty stomach, right? That's when suddenly absolutely everything looks so tasty—and you just can't resist! Well, just as you shouldn't go shopping on an empty stomach, the same is true for partying: Don't arrive at a party hungry. Eat a small meal or some healthy snacks beforehand, and you'll be less likely to overindulge. Also, make the right choices! Part of maintaining positive thinking is choosing correctly. Now I know that *you* know that eating that cheese ball instead of a carrot is not the right choice, but don't kill yourself for having one or two! But there are other good decisions to make: you can choose dark chocolate over brownies, or a fresh-fruit sorbet over a creamy ice cream.

KEEPING UP WITH WATER TIPS

Water—especially high-quality filtered water—is your best friend. The standard of eight glasses of water a day is a good one to stick to. Start with one first thing in the morning and then right before and in between meals. Actually, it's best not to sip too much more than a cup during meals, because it affects digestion and how we burn fat. As for other drinks, try sticking closer to juices in their natural state—which would be unprocessed. In fact, stay away from most, if not all, processed food and drinks!

Guidelines for Exercise

DO SOME FORM OF CARDIO EXERCISE
AT LEAST THREE DAYS A WEEK

Ideally you should have at least thirty minutes of cardio at least three days a week. Walking briskly for even one to two hours a week (fifteen to twenty minutes a day) will certainly help, but more is ideal. However, if you don't like walking, any activity that makes your heart work harder (riding a bike, dancing, playing a sport) will be enough, as long as you do it long enough and often enough. Remember that thirty minutes of moderate-intensity activity a day is great as a starting point, but not an upper limit. If you can exercise for longer—and harder—you will reap the most benefits.

Also, everyone needs to exercise at the correct heart rate to get the most cardiovascular benefits and to stay safe. This heart rate is called your target or training heart rate; it is the rate you want your heart beating at during vigorous exercise. Most fitness experts advise exercising at between 55 percent and 85 percent of your maximum heart rate for optimal benefits. The way to find your target heart rate is to follow this formula:

Take your age and subtract it from 220. Now multiply that number by .55. Also multiply the same number by .85. The answers will give you your ideal heart-rate range.

Here is an example: Elizabeth is 40 years old.

$$220 - 40 = 180$$
$$180 \times .55 = 99$$
$$180 \times .85 = 153$$

Elizabeth should have a heart rate above 99 while exercising to get any cardiovascular benefit. But she should never allow her heart rate to go above 153 while exercising. A pulse somewhere in the middle will be the best for optimal performance and in the safest range.

Another way to test that is very easy is to see if you can hold a conversation while exercising (this is sometimes called the talk test): If you are slightly out of breath but able to speak and breathe deeply, then this is aerobic activity that is good for fat burning. If you are panting and out of breath, and not able to speak for any length of time, then you are giving your heart a workout, but also burning more glucose than fat (anaerobic exercise). I recommend doing both types of exercise: aerobic and anaerobic. So let's say you are dancing to some great salsa: dance within your training zone, and then halfway through add in a vigorous five minutes to get you really sweating, and then bring the movements back to a more relaxed flow. This applies to any type of exercise. No need to get more complicated than this unless you are doing some serious athletic training.

The following table shows estimated target heart rates for different ages. Look for the age category closest to yours, then read across to find your target heart rate.

TARGET HEART RATES FOR DIFFERENT AGES

Age	Target HR Zone 50–85%	Average Maximum Heart Rate 100%
20 years	100–170 beats per minute	200 beats per minute
25 years	98–166 beats per minute	195 beats per minute
30 years	95–162 beats per minute	190 beats per minute
35 years	93–157 beats per minute	185 beats per minute
40 years	90–153 beats per minute	180 beats per minute
45 years	88–149 beats per minute	175 beats per minute
50 years	85–145 beats per minute	170 beats per minute
55 years	83–140 beats per minute	165 beats per minute
60 years	80–136 beats per minute	160 beats per minute
65 years	78–132 beats per minute	155 beats per minute
70 years	75–128 beats per minute	150 beats per minute

Source: http://www.americanheart.org

Note: Your maximum heart rate is about 220 minus your age. The figures above are averages, so use them as general guidelines.

Fitting in an exercise routine is not always easy, right? After all, we're swamped; between work, kids, and everything else, who has time to go hang out in a gym? Well, if this sounds like you, let me make a suggestion: try walking more! Here are some tips for fitting walking into your schedule.

AT HOME

▶ Get up thirty minutes earlier and take a stroll (take the dog and/or your hubby, too!).

▶ Walk up and down the stairs a certain number of times a day.

▶ Get up and walk around—even when you're watching TV.

AT WORK

▶ We're so used to door-to-door commutes—but if you take a train or bus to work, you can get off a stop or two early and walk the rest of the way.

▶ If you're driving, park your car in the space that is the farthest away and walk to the office.

▶ These days, everyone's doing the IM, text messaging, and phone thing—even when we're talking to someone in the next office. If you need to speak to somebody in the office, walk over to them!

▶ Use your lunchtime to take a walk around the block.

▶ Whenever possible, use the stairs instead of the elevator.

MAKE IT A FAMILY AFFAIR

▶ Make each kid feel special by devoting time for one walk a week with each child so he/she can have some private "mommy time."

▶ Walk your children to school or day care.

▶ Walk to the park and back on weekends.

▶ Find walking tours and interesting sites to explore.

▶ Take a romantic sunset (or early-morning) stroll with your beloved.

With *amigos* (your friends!):

▶ Plan walks with your friends—so you can catch up and work out.

▶ Instead of getting donuts and coffee with your pals, pick up those sneakers and walk together.

CHALLENGE YOUR BODY AND
PICK UP A NEW SPORT OR DANCE FOR EVERY YEAR

Most people fall off the exercise wagon simply because of boredom. It's inevitable that following a routine can get repetitive and boring. Also, the results of cardio exercise will taper off after time if you don't challenge your body and reach for higher goals. That's why it's important to introduce new, fun exercises into your routine, or pick up a new sport or dance that you've always wanted to try. Salsa dancing has so many benefits: it's a low-impact exercise (so you don't have the possibility of high-impact-related knee and back injuries), it boosts physical endurance, and it increases your range of motion. And—on top of this—it's incredibly sensual and expressive, and a lot of fun. For me it's one of those wonderful (and rare!) marriages where you're doing something great for your body while having a fabulous time. For this reason, it's one of the best ways to get into shape.

The bottom line is this: Any physical activity is great! Whether it be walking, swimming, running, hiking, skating, or skiing, the most important attribute your exercise of choice must have is stick-to-itiveness! In other words, you've got to find activities you like, and do them regularly. If you keep them up, you will not only burn calories and feel better, you'll also improve your metabolism and ultimately benefit your overall health.

COMPLEMENT CARDIO WITH RESISTANCE TRAINING

Weight training burns some calories (for example, a 130-pound female training hard for twenty minutes burns about 117 calories; a 150-pound female doing moderate training burns about 68 calories in the same period), but running or cycling will certainly burn more. Remember: Ideal workouts combine cardio and resistive exercise.

When you're in your mid to late twenties, you start to lose muscle as part of the natural aging process. This means that the amount of calories you need each day starts to decrease and it becomes easier to gain weight. However, regular strength training can help to decrease this loss of lean muscle tissue and even replace some that has been lost already. Many trainers and doctors say that strength training will increase lean body mass, decrease fat mass, and increase resting metabolic rate (a measurement of the amount of calories burned per day).

Resistance training also helps with bone strength and the fight against osteoporosis. In older women, strength training can greatly help their ability to perform basic physical functions—from getting up from a chair, to walking, to climbing up stairs.

With weight training, you will achieve the same results if you choose a higher number of reps with low resistance, or more weight with fewer reps—but this also depends on your current fitness level. In the beginning, though, you should use lighter weights so that you can finish twelve to fifteen repetitions of each exercise for two sets. Then, when two to three sets of fifteen repetitions is no longer challenging, you can increase the weight so that you can handle twelve reps but it's still challenging. As you become more conditioned, you can handle higher weights with fewer reps per set. Using higher weights—or more resistance—will greatly overload the muscle, which will in turn get you stronger quicker, while adding more lean mass to your frame. Also, your resting metabolism will increase, which translates into burning more calories at rest. Furthermore, you should vary your resistance exercise so that you engage more total muscle fibers while doing them. Squats or leg presses, bench presses, lat pull-downs, and overhead presses, for example, all help build muscle more quickly than isolated, one-joint exercises will. It is best not to do resistance training daily, but rather every other day, in order to give your muscles time to rest, repair, and build between workouts.

GET THE PROPER NUTRITION FOR YOUR WORKOUT

A preworkout snack will help you by giving you the energy you need for your workout. The best snack should be a combination of proteins, unsaturated fats, and complex carbohydrates. If you eat foods that are high in fats, on the other hand, you will feel sluggish because your body takes longer to digest them. Ideally, your preworkout snack should total less than 300 calories. Fruit, nuts, or rice cakes and organic peanut butter are good choices.

While you're working out, and sweating away sodium, potassium, and magnesium, you're losing electrolytes, which are responsible for muscle contractions as well as regulating the fluid balance in and out of your cells. Therefore, it's important to keep yourself hydrated throughout your exercise program.

According to the American College of Sports Medicine's guidelines, you should be drinking the following amounts of water before, during, and after your workouts:

▶ Before—about 16 ounces, about 2 hours beforehand

▶ During—5 to 10 ounces every 20 minutes

▶ After—at least 2 large glasses of water (between 16 and 24 ounces)

After working out, your body's energy levels are substantially depleted and must be restocked. This is also the time that your muscles—which are getting ready for your next exercise session—begin their recovery process. Because of this, it's important for you to ingest protein and carbohydrates within forty-five minutes.

Other Considerations for the Long Haul

- ✔ Limit your intake of hydrogenated fats, which contain harmful trans-fatty acids. These are found in many chips, French fries, margarine, and cookies. Instead, use healthy oils like olive, corn, and soy.

- ✔ Make smart choices if fast food is your only option. Choose fresh fruit or salad plates, whole wheat bread or tortillas, small portions—even kids' sizes, if possible (but no supersizing!)—choose grilled meat or fish (no fried dishes), and please leave those sugar- and fat-packed special sauces behind.

- ✔ Decrease your consumption of red meat, and try replacing it with turkey or chicken—or fish (or even vegetables!). There are so many ways to replace meat in recipes and enjoy a terrific menu of dishes with less fat and more flavor!

- ✔ Try eating less refined grains—white rice, white flour, and products made from them. Instead reach for brown rice, wild rice, healthful grains, and whole-wheat flour.

- ✔ Lessen your consumption of full-fat products like whole milk, cheese, sour cream, and ice cream. Try using these products with less or no fat, or reducing the amount you eat. Light coconut milk, for example, offers you a nice creamy alternative—and Latin American cheeses, like Mexico's *queso fresco* (literally, fresh cheese), with just a dollop atop black beans, corn tortillas, vegetables, or whatever you'd like can offer you plenty of flavor—even in small amounts—and much less fat than what you usually reach for.

- ✔ Also, reach for chicken stock—homemade, of course, is best, but you can find excellent-quality organic chicken stock on many shelves these days—as a seasoning ingredient instead of fats.

- ✔ Avoid artificial flavor enhancers, which generally have a lot of chemicals like MSG and hydrolyzed proteins; do use spices and herbs for flavoring with additional benefits. Also, use sea salt or kosher salt instead of table salt.

- ✔ Limit your intake of sweets and sugary drinks, like sodas and many juices.

EPILOGUE

At this point, I want you to pause for a moment of reflection. Consider the following questions:

1. Do I feel better?

2. Are some of my aches and pains remedied?

3. Am I sleeping better?

4. Is my mental mood more positive?

5. Has my sex life improved?

6. Do I want to continue feeling like this?

If the Hot Latin Diet has helped you answer positively to any one of these questions, it has positively impacted how you are living. Take these lessons and make them your mantra for the rest of your life. Remember the following:

1. Eat good food (Latin powerfoods).

2. Practice portion control.

3. Do plenty of physical activity.

4 Understand that quick fixes are not the answer.

5 Remember it's okay to make a mistake.

WE'VE ONLY JUST BEGUN

I guess I'm dating myself by quoting the title of the 1970s Carpenters' song, but I mean it! Though this is the end of this book, it's part of such an exciting beginning. I know that old habits are tough to bury, but I also know that you're making an effort—and working hard to achieve your goals. And why shouldn't you? Life is short; we've got to make the most of it today—and every day. Part of this means taking great care of ourselves so that we can all be happy, feel great, and look hot!

So, my friend, my heartfelt thoughts are with you as you continue to thrive on this Hot Latin Diet lifestyle. So instead of saying good-bye, I'm going to say *hasta luego*, see you later!

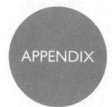

QUESTIONS AND ANSWERS
FROM THE HOT LATIN DIET CHEFS

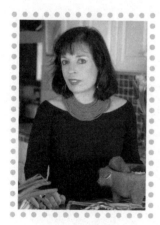

Chef Zarela Martínez

How do you describe a woman who has brought so many people's awareness about such a profound and rich cuisine to a new level of understanding and respect?

Zarela Martínez's life is proof that creative energy has no bounds. Zarela, who continually draws on her Mexican childhood for ideas and inspiration—as well as frequent visits back to her native country—is one of today's most accomplished chefs and restaurateurs. But there's so much more: she's also a noted educator on the topic of Mexican food, through both her restaurant and her PBS television series, and online at www.zarela.com. Since 1987, New York City has been graced with her restaurant, Zarela, which boasts not only rave reviews and a devoted following but also a plethora of recipes from the rich regions of Mexico. Her public television series, *Zarela! La Cocina Veracruzana*, teaches about the unique Mediterranean- and African-accented regional cooking of the state of Veracruz. The author of three cookbooks, an active speaker, and a teacher—as well as chef and restaurateur—Zarela has also created her own line of Mexican-inspired home furnishings, called Zarela Casa.

Chef Zarela Martínez's Recipes Included Here

- Ejotes con Huevo (String Beans with Egg)—Breakfast

- Ensalada Girasol (Sunflower Salad)—Lunch

- Espinacas (Wilted Spinach)—Snack

Q AND A WITH CHEF ZARELA MARTÍNEZ

Q: Zarela, through your restaurant, cookbooks, television shows, and now your Web site, you've played a key role in introducing many people to the richness of Mexican cooking. What advice can you give people who are just being introduced to your cuisine?

A: It's very important to have a well-stocked pantry with all the ingredients you're going to use—like chipotles en adobo, Mexican oregano, pickled jalapeños, and so on.

Q: I notice that you use a lot of chipotle, which is one of our Hot Latin powerfoods. Tell me a bit about that.

A: I find that smoky chipotle chiles are universally liked, and my favorite way to use them is in an easy-to-make and versatile chipotle paste made with canned chipotle chiles in adobo, which are widely available now. The paste keeps well.

I also want to encourage people to try ingredients just entering the U.S. market—herbs like *hoja santa* (an anise-flavor leaf), avocado leaves used to make *barbacoas* (Mexican-style barbecue dishes in which the leaves actually permeate the food and add wonderful flavor), and old standbys like tomatillos.

Q: What do you make with tomatillos, another one of our seven Latin powerfoods?

A: Oh—there are so many things, but you can make a real simple sauce with raw tomatillos, onion, jalapeños, cilantro, and garlic, and just like the chipotle paste, you will find so many ways to use it—on top of grilled fish, chicken, meat, and more.

Q: When you're creating a dish, what are some of your considerations?

A: I think of taste in terms of layers of flavor and textures so that the flavors hit your palate at different times as you chew. You have to keep your palate excited all the time. I go to the farmer's market every week and like to use vegetables and fruits in season. I look forward to my first cherry or pomegranate of the year and anxiously await the appearance of the first ramps (wild leeks) in spring and parsley root in the fall.

Q: Zarela, you're in such great shape. What do you do to help you stay so fit and looking so great?

A: I eat well! And I finish my meals early in the day—we usually eat dinner at about five thirty or six p.m.—and I do a lot of yoga.

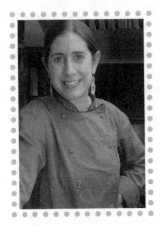

Chef Sue Torres

How fitting that the name of the chef and restaurateur Sue Torres's first restaurant is Sueños, which means dreams in Spanish. This passionate and tenacious New York native is certainly making her dreams come true; her interpretations of the cuisine she's been endlessly in love with have been delighting many old and newfound fans. A graduate of the Culinary Institute of America, Torres first became enamored with Mexico's culinary treasures when she became sous-chef at New York's Arizona 206 and Arizona Café. Torres, anxious to solidify her education of Mexican cuisine at its source, traveled to study with the Mexican-cooking authority and cookbook writer Diana Kennedy, who taught her the roots of this country's fare. By learning the fundamentals, and combining that knowledge with both her education and professional experience, Torres was able to apply her creativity and innovation to produce her own contemporary versions. By the start of 2003, after serving stints as chef and executive chef at New York City's highly acclaimed Rocking Horse Café in Hell's Kitchen, Torres was ready to translate her fascination with this cuisine into the creation of her own Mexican restaurants. Sueños and her newest restaurant, Los Dados (which means dice in Spanish), reflect in both menu and décor how Torres so deftly combines colors, fresh flavors, and a variety of textures.

Chef Sue Torres's Recipes Included Here

- Migas (Mexican-Style Breakfast)

- Grilled Salmon with Green Sauce and Tomatillo-Pineapple Salsa—Lunch

- Fruit with Chile de Árbol and Lime Juice—Snack

- Grilled Vegetables with Cilantro Pesto—Snack

- Coriander-Crusted Chicken Breast with Grilled Chipotle-Sparked Potatoes and Mustard Greens—Dinner

Q AND A WITH CHEF SUE TORRES

Q: Sue, you know I'm in love with your Cilantro Pesto (I just had some now on top of a piece of whole-wheat toast!), and it's not just because it's one of our Hot Latin powerfoods! What are your favorite pestos, salsas, and sauces?

A: Cilantro pesto is now my favorite. I grew up on basil pesto, so this is a variation on the traditional basil pesto. My favorite salsa is salsa verde, made with tomatillos, garlic, onions, cilantro, and serrano chiles. And I also really like the smoky, fiery flavors of red salsa, too!

Q: Your dishes are intense combinations of flavors and colors. Tell me a bit about your inspiration for creating new dishes.

A: What's in season—and what looks good! I go to the market and see what's there, and then I let availability dictate my ingredients—like beautiful tomatoes in summer, and great acorn squash in the fall—and then I make them Mexican style. Also, I cook what I like to eat! Sometimes I'll get inspired at midnight one night, and put the dish on my menu the next day!

Q: We have your recipe for Coriander-Crusted Chicken. Tell me about why you chose coriander.

A: Coriander is one of the most beautiful aromatics! It adds great flavor *and* texture—I love coriander! I'd put it on bread if I could! Coriander is perfect on the chicken we have here—but also on tuna, venison, and filet mignon.

Q: I know you enjoy eating a lot, yet it doesn't show. What are some of your tricks for staying in such great shape?

A: Eating right—the right foods at the right time. Exercise—yoga and cardio. I ride my bike around New York City, and I work with a trainer who knows me, knows what I like, and knows my body—and how to push me.

Q: What do you recommend to someone who is just getting started with a new diet?

A: You have to have a positive outlook—you have to be inspired! You have to say to yourself, "I've got this great idea and I'm going to make it work." You have to start with a clean slate. Also, with exercise, you have to find something that you want to do so that you can stick to it. So if you don't like jogging, don't do it! You might want to try a couple of things. Don't give up until you try a few things. There's a fighter in everyone—you just have to find it!

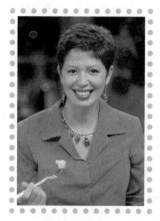

Chef Daisy Martínez

You can smell the perfume of fresh-baked bread, combined with that of a myriad of spices and herbs that dance together to give depth to every plate that she prepares, whether you're reading her cookbooks or watching her on television. Growing up in the enchanted kitchens of her Puerto Rican *abuelas* (grandmothers)—as well as her mom's—certainly inspired Daisy Martínez. Though she started her career as a model and actress, her husband knew her deep love for entertaining and cooking, and gave her the gift of furthering her culinary education at the French Culinary Institute. Daisy, whose credits include working on the set of PBS's *Lidia's Italian-American Kitchen* as a prep-kitchen chef, as well as managing a small catering business (The Passionate Palate), which she continues to operate, is also quite active outside the kitchen. She regularly visits schools as a featured speaker and participates in many philanthropic events. Daisy's embrace of her cultural roots, and her broad knowledge of Latin cuisine, are highlighted in *Daisy Cooks!*, her highly rated PBS television program and popular cookbook, for which she is an IACP nominee and winner of the Best Latino Cuisine Cookbook in the World from the Gourmand World Cookbook Awards, as well as on her Web site, www.daisymartínez.com/.

Chef Daisy Martínez's Recipes Included Here

- Torrejas (Latin-Style French Toast)—Breakfast

- Quinoa Risotto Primavera—Lunch

- Soursop-Mango Blush Batida—Snack

- Pan-Seared Red Snapper with Grapefruit-Avocado Salsa—Dinner

Q AND A WITH CHEF DAISY MARTÍNEZ

Q: Daisy, on your television show, on your Web site, and in your books, you "welcome" people into the world of Latin cooking. What advice do you have for people who are just getting introduced to the flavors of your cooking?

A: Contrary to what your mother told you, I'm all about playing with your food! My recipes are more of a guideline than a strict follow-this-to-the-letter rule (which, in my humble opinion, only applies to baking). So I would say that you should play with different kinds of heat, and acids, like citrus—oranges, limes, lemons, grapefruits—as well as vinegars, and try different flavors: melt anchovy in a sauce, or add a teaspoon of olive tapenade! Playing with these different flavors makes it more interesting. When people ask me about Latin cooking, I want to make sure they understand that it's fun, vibrant, sexy, and sassy.

Q: What are your key pantry ingredients?

A: I always have *sofrito* (a traditional base to many Latin-style dishes) in the freezer, and all the components (onions, garlic, bell peppers, and cilantro) in the vegetable bin, and this will help you working moms get from zero to a healthy dinner for your family in forty-five minutes!

Q: What are the dishes you most typically cook for your family?

A: There's nothing that I don't make! We, my three gorgeous sons and beautiful daughter, and my husband, eat all kinds of stuff—and I don't cook just Latin food. Actually, my husband is Italian, so I cook a lot of Italian, but also many different Asian (all kinds of stir-fries) and French dishes. The aspect of nutrition is always important—my husband is a physician, so he's just as interested in healthy eating.

I always make sure we have soup or salad (gotta get their greens!) with red onion and basil, and shaved fennel. I go to the market and get ideas. Also, I make different dressings using flavored oils, flavored vinegars, and citrus—like grapefruit with honey and olive oil.

And dinner always consists of a protein, a vegetable, and a starch. Dessert—especially in the summer—is fresh fruit with yogurt. We also like to roast pineapples on the grill—that's good eating! If the children grow up with that, that's what they'll turn to!

My kids eat well because that's what they were taught. They have sophisticated palates—they've been taught that they don't have to finish all their food, but that they have to taste everything on their plate!

Q: You used to be a professional model and actress and are now on television and always looking great. What advice can you give women who are trying to keep their figures or get their figures back?

A: Walk, walk, walk! Walking and stretching is the everywoman workout.

I live in a gorgeous old three-story Victorian house, so I'm up and down the stairs. Also, I have a market one block away, and another four blocks away. I'll walk to the one that's four blocks away, because that's a way to get in my exercise. I deny myself nothing—but everything in moderation! And I don't feel like I'm cheating. If I taste one or two mouthfuls, I satisfy my experience. . . .

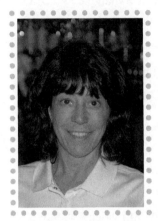

Chef Xiomara Ardolina

Fans in California have touted the talents of the Cuban-born chef and restaurateur Xiomara Ardolina for a long time, and why wouldn't they? After all, Xiomara's charm, energy, humor, and incredible culinary savvy have been blessing the West Coast for close to two decades—and in two different culinary languages: first in French, and now in Nuevo Latino. Xiomara came to the United States from Cuba when she was just thirteen years old. You could say that the restaurant business is in her blood; as a child she became fascinated with the industry as she watched her godparents run their restaurant. Years later, in New York, she received her training, and then took her show on the road to California, where she's become the proud chef and owner of two restaurants. Though she first became well known for her talents with French cuisine, she has now developed her own brand of Nuevo Latino cooking. Ardolina's menus are drawn principally from her Cuban heritage, but are additionally infused with her French flair. The results, as Southern Californians know, are magnificent! In her restaurant Café Atlantic, and now in Xiomara, this chef proves again and again that anyone can—and should—fall in love with Latin flavors.

Chef Xiomara Ardolina's Recipes Included Here

Ceviche—Lunch

- Huevos Campesinos (Farmer-Style Eggs) with Red Bell Pepper Sauce—Breakfast

- Xiomara Salad—Dinner

- Shrimp with a Mango-Ginger Sauce—Dinner

- Churrasco (Marinated Skirt Steak)—Dinner

- Bistec Empanizado (Citrus and Spice-Marinated and Breaded Steak)—Dinner

Q AND A WITH CHEF XIOMARA ARDOLINA

Q: Your transition from French cuisine back to your native flavors is an interesting one—and it seems like your recipes represent the best of both worlds. When you're creating a recipe, what are your primary considerations?

A: Because I'm Cuban, I like to integrate Latin flavors in whatever I'm making, and I try to cook everything with its own juices. I try not to use too much butter, because bringing out the flavors we have is so easy! You can season with a *sofrito* of onion, garlic, cumin, and oregano, which are actually ingredients in Mediterranean cooking, too.

Q: Are there other cuisines that you especially enjoy cooking, and/or eating?

A: Italian! I love Italian cuisine—our food is so different! I love pasta with basil and fresh tomato, but I can't put that on my Nuevo Latino menu! I also really like Greek cuisine—cooking with mint or lime; I don't have a favorite. For example, sometimes for a barbecue, I'll make Greek-style hamburgers on pita with sour cream and mint.

Q: What advice can you give women as they try your recipes?

A: It's all about flavors—and marinating! Like I just told my daughter, who's going to Boston College, marinating adds so much flavor. Take chicken, for example—just smash some garlic, add some fresh lime juice and fresh orange juice, salt, and pepper, and marinate for between twenty minutes and an hour. Just giving it a bit of flavor at the beginning makes a huge difference. Then add rice, or pasta, and a salad, and you're in great shape! You can also marinate fish—but not for too long, because it will "cook" in the acids of the citrus juices—and meat.

Q: What suggestions do you have with regard to women who are starting to diet?

A: Don't give up flavor! People think that when they eat diet food it has to be plain and tasteless; you can put so much flavor in your food without fat. Even just olive oil, lime, and salt add a lot of flavor! I love bread, but I say stay away from bread—and too much starch. You should watch your portions. Have your vegetables, and have a piece of chicken, meat, or fish.

Q: Though you're surrounded by food all the time, you're obviously in great shape. Do you exercise?

A: I watch what I eat—and I run! I run five miles every day, and I also play tennis and golf.

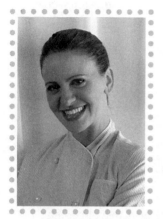

Chef Michelle Bernstein

Whether she's on NBC's *Today* show, duking it out on the Food Network's *Iron Chef*, winning yet another James Beard Federation nomination, or toiling in the kitchen of Michy's, her highly acclaimed Miami restaurant, one thing is for sure: Chef Michelle Bernstein is a role model for any aspiring chef. Her drive, as well as her unique cultural background as a Jewish-Latino woman, guides her deep passion for food and the art of its preparation. Once teased—because of her svelte stature—for being a lightweight in the restaurant she interned in, this former ballerina turned professional chef, restaurateur, television star, consulting chef for Delta Airlines, and now cookbook author, has most certainly proven that she is a heavyweight in many arenas. Recognized repeatedly for her many talents, Chef Bernstein was given a doctorate in Culinary Arts from Johnson & Wales University, was named one of *Latina* magazine's top women in 2006, was given the Philanthropic Award of South Florida, as well as the Glass Ceiling award from the Jewish Federation, and was named one of the Top Jewish Women in America by the Jewish Women International Federation. Bernstein, who continues to dazzle us with her multifaceted endeavors, is currently expanding her role as restaurateur, and will have her first cookbook published by Houghton Mifflin.

Chef Michelle Bernstein's Recipes Included Here

- Spicy Frittata, Tomato Salad—Breakfast

- Grilled Tuna Niçoise—Lunch

- Spiced-Up Hummus—Snack

- Star Anise and Ginger-Spiced Chicken with Roast Calabaza and Corn—Dinner

Q AND A WITH CHEF MICHELLE BERNSTEIN

Q: You have such a wonderful way of combining different flavors—as in your chicken dinner, wonderfully spiced with star anise, ginger, cumin, fennel, and more. What are your guiding principles in combining spices?

A: My only guiding principles are my sense of taste and smell—through memory and travels. Every once in a while I'm surprised by flavor combinations, but I have profiles in my mind and memory banks—thanks to all the traveling and eating I've done—of what works and what doesn't work.

Q: You've also combined many Mediterranean flavors with your Latin ones. What are some of your other favorite culinary influences?

A: If I could tell you all of my influences it would fill up many pages! I've been lucky to travel a lot, and have been invited to places as far away and as varied as Malaysia, Korea, France, and Peru (to give cooking classes and gastronomic tours). To be honest, it's such a vast experience, and every time I go to a new country I find a whole new wonderful world of culture and flavor.

Q: Do you always eat what you cook? Do you ever do takeout?

A: We do everything, but I normally don't enjoy my own cooking! I'm hypercritical of my own food, especially in the restaurant, where

I'm definitely my own worst critic! But I'll eat almost anything—and I love it when others cook for me; whether it's Chinese takeout or one of my favorite tapas restaurants, I really enjoy eating other people's cooking. I greatly appreciate all the work that goes into preparing a meal.

Q: You've stopped dancing professionally, but still have the figure of a ballet dancer. What are some of your eating habits?

A: I eat in moderation. And if I cheat, I make sure I'm disciplined after that. It's hard to not dip into everything all day long—it's hard for any chef! But my husband and I walk and bike quite a bit, and sometimes I do weight training. I am very active—I'm always running or doing something physical, whether it's for work or in my garden.

Q: What do you recommend to women who are starting to diet?

A: The best thing is to decide you're going to change your lifestyle, but not that you're on a diet. Say, "I've decided I want to eat better!" We psyche ourselves out when we say "diet"—don't think of that nasty four-letter word!

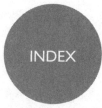

INDEX

Sodium, in fast food, 2

Soursop-Mango Blush Batida (Shake), 132

South Beach Diet, 27–29

Soybean oil, 71

Spiced-Up Hummus, 130

Spices (*see* Herbs and spices)

Spicy Frittata, Tomato Salad, 97–98

Spinach, 16, 65

    Espinacas (Wilted Spinach), 131

Spirit, guidelines for the, 158–63

Spirulina bars, 169–70

Sports drinks, 72

Star Anise and Ginger-Spiced Chicken with Roast

    Calabaza and Corn, 103–5

Starches (complex carbohydrates), 12, 62, 66

Steward, H. Leighton, 30

Stress, 59

    dealing with, 159–60, 176

Stretching, 161

Stroke, 21, 24

Sucrose, 56, 67, 68

Sugar alcohols, 56, 67

Sugar Busters Diet, 30–31

Sugars

    content, 67–69

    on food labels, 55, 67

    forms of, 56

    recommended daily intake, 68–69

Sustainable Agriculture Research and Education Program

    (USDA), 22

Sweeteners, artificial, 56, 67

Target heart rate, 177–79

Tarnower, Herman, 25

3-Hour Diet, 32–33

Tiradito, 21

Toasted Garbanzo Beans, 110–11

Toasted Pumpkin Seeds (Pepitas), 153

Tomatillo-Pineapple Salsa, 121–22

Tomatillos, 3, 16, 64, 164

    described, 12

Tomatoes, 14, 16, 64

Torrejas, 115

    recipe for, 119–20

Torres, Sue, 5, 109, 114, 115, 121, 137, 148, 192–94

Toxic metals, 14

Trans fat, 39, 55, 56, 70–73

Triglycerides, 21

Trout, 15, 17

Tubers (*see* Grains, tubers, and nuts)

Tuna Niçoise, Grilled, 99–100

Turkey, 15, 18, 22

Unsaturated fat, 55

Utensil size, 166

Vegetable oils, 72

Vegetables, Grilled, with Cilantro Pesto,

    148–50

Vegetables and chiles (*see also* Dinner recipes; Lunch

      recipes; Snack recipes)

    benefits of, 19–20

    categories of, 14, 16

    as fiber source, 76

    glycemic index ratings for, 64–65

Vegetarians/vegans, 27, 32, 74, 91–92, 165

Vitamins

    A, 12, 19, 70

    B_6, 19, 22

    B_{12}, 22

    C, 12, 19, 20, 77

    D, 38, 70

    E, 20, 22, 70

    K, 70

Waist-hip ratio (WHR), 84–85

Walking, 177, 179–80

Walnuts, 71

Water intake, 38, 39, 72, 76–77, 113, 177, 183

Watermelon, 16, 64

Weight chart, according to frame, 82

Weight gain, top eight factors contributing to,

    58–62

Weight training, 181–83

Weight Watchers, 31–32

Wheat bran, 76

Whey, 56

WHR (waist-hip ratio), 84–85